Journey Forward:

 For more information, address Two Crabs And A Lion Publishers, 4000 W. 106th Street, Ste 125-148, Carmel, IN 46032

Two Crabs And A Lion books may be purchased for educational, business, or sales promotional use. For information, please email 2crabs1lion@gmail.com.

FIRST EDITION

Designed by Keva M. Richardson

Library of Congress Cataloging-in-Publication Data

Names: Henderson-Wilson, Robin
Turner, Nathaniel A.
Title: Journey Forward: How to Use Journaling to Envision and Manifest the Life You Always Wanted
Description: First Edition. | Carmel, Indiana: Two Crabs And A Lion, 2021
Identifiers: LCCN 2021912450 (print) | ISBN 978-0-9895879-9-0 (print) |ISBN 978-1-7352666-2-6 (e-book)
Subjects: LSCH: Self-Help Techniques | Mind & Body | BISAC: HEALTH & FITNESS / Mental Health | SELF-HELP / Journaling | BODY, MIND & SPIRIT / Mindfulness & Meditation

ACKNOWLEDGEMENT

You knew and nurtured God's purpose for me long before I was aware of His plan for me. There are no words that can properly capture my depth of gratitude. Your presence is both missed and felt daily. This one is for you, Mommy!

Robin E. Henderson-Wilson

PREFACE BY NATHANIEL A. TURNER

Are you familiar with the word "voluntold"? If you are, it's the simplest way to explain how and why this book exists.

If you aren't familiar with the word "voluntold" by some good fortune, let me say congratulations. Hopefully, having no previous knowledge of the word means you have yet to get introduced to a life where you often don't get the opportunity to choose for yourself if you want to volunteer for a cause alleged to be voluntary participation only.

Voluntold is a word that means instead of volunteering for something, someone assigns a task to you. Being voluntold is precisely how this book was born. I know Dr. Henderson-Wilson would prefer not to admit to it, but that's pretty much how *Journey Forward* came to be the book it is today. Dr. Henderson-Wilson voluntold me to do it!

A couple of years ago, I shared some of my forward journal entries with her, and after reading them, she first recommended that I share them with others. She found them encouraging, inspiring, routinely comical, and a way to stay authentically mindful of the call all humans have to live a life of great purpose.

Later she recommended that I compile fifty-two entries, write reflections and action statements for each entry, and then publish them in a book. I won't even bother telling you about the next series of "recommendations," i.e., an online course, a podcast, the creation of a journaling forward community, and the like. I'll merely say stay tuned for what else Dr. Henderson-Wilson voluntold me to do.

This scenario described above is what is meant by the word voluntold precisely. However, not to be outdone believing turnabout is fair play, I voluntold Dr. Henderson-Wilson to share in the book's publication. To be a book, I voluntold Dr. Henderson-Wilson that she would have to write the reflections and action statements she thought we needed to include in a book.

Before being voluntold to share my journal, I wrote privately. I journaled to support my mental health, lend myself a spiritual helping hand, and even give myself a swift kick in the butt. Beyond believing I can and should do more with my life now, the journaling forward first served to help with my mental health as I suffer from depression.

I'm no longer afraid to admit I get depressed. So many times, depression takes me to a deep, melancholy, oft excruciating dark place. One way that I discovered that helps treat my depression is to write forward in my journal.

When I started keeping a traditional journal, I often felt more anxious and depressed after writing in it. On the rare occasions that I felt better, I felt only slightly better after writing in my journal than before I started writing.

In retrospect, it's no surprise that I didn't feel better after having written. Because, in the beginning, I wrote about things that didn't go well, people who angered and disappointed me, and all the seemingly untenable trials and tribulations of life. So for me, this form of traditional journaling was, without question, counterproductive.

One day, after writing an unquestionably negative journal entry, I remembered thinking what a waste of time to relive undesirable moments. Getting things out of one's system is one thing, but that should not be the only outcome I get from journaling.

Then I thought! What if instead of recalling and then reliving on paper or electronic document a moment I disdained, I instead imagined my best life, and I wrote about that? What if I wrote about my best life, my imagined desired life, first thing in the morning before I did anything else? Even when I have an unfortunate experience, what if, I write about that experience in the past tense? What if I envisioned a moment in the future when that experience will only be a memory of how far I've come professionally or how far I've grown as a person?

Over the years, I've learned neuroscience and psychiatry support this exercise of journaling forward. Nevertheless, the cliff notes non-neuroscientist and psychiatrist version of the journaling forward story is the brain does not distinguish between prior memories and future ruminations.

Journaling forward allows me to create future hopeful moments and pleasant dreamt chronicles. Thus, journaling forward is essentially self-programming my mind for a type of enjoyable time travel.

Rather than dwelling on past events that saddened me and left me profoundly depressed or worse, I wrote about how I imagined living my best life. Also, when confronted with a situation that didn't go as desired in reality, I wrote about a future event featuring the same circumstances where the virtual outcome was the one I wanted.

In the past many years of journaling forward, I've found myself less depressed. Moreover, it's helped me do a better job managing anxiety often associated with a pending bout of depression. In short, journaling forward allows me to reduce the usually engulfing and long-lingering effects of anxiety and depression.

And there have been surprising bonuses from journaling forward. A number of the things I wrote about manifested themselves in my life.

From writing books, giving a TED Talk, being invited to keynote public and private engagements, and being featured in national publications and media outlets throughout the county, journaling forward has been a fantastic way to keep me living in the moment. Forward journaling has helped me keep my sanity. It also motivates me to remain faithful to my PVP (personal value proposition). More often, I now live my life with joy on purpose so that daily I may help, serve, and make sure others know that their life matters.

So that's how we got here. That's why 'Journey Forward' now exists. Thanks to the persistent nudge of a lifelong friend. Thanks to being "voluntold" to share what helps me deal with depression, restrain overwhelming despair caused by the events like the Pandemic, and manage the daily trials and tribulations of life, 'Journey Forward' is a book today.

I hope that you find some value in 'Journey Forward.' Moreover, I hope that you will now journal forward the life you always imagined living too.

Table of Contents

Journey Forward:

INTRODUCTION BY ROBIN E. HENDERSON-WILSON

Dear Journal

What would you do if one day you open an email from a life-long friend and that e-mail begins like this..."Dear Journal"? Well, that's exactly how this story begins. First, I received an e-mail that began, "Dear Journal."

I kept reading and discovered a fascinating concept, forward journaling. I must admit that initially, I thought my friend had lost his mind. It only took reading a few sentences, though, to recognize my friend had not lost his mind. But instead, he was using his mind to craft the future he envisioned for himself, his loved ones, and, quite frankly, the world.

World-renowned author, speaker, catalyst for change, and most importantly, Naeem's father, Nathaniel Turner, gifts us insights into how he propels himself into action every day. Before Nate changed how grown-ups across the globe, "adult," he began by casting a vision for his own life. He envisioned an image of himself not bound by current circumstances but open to the world of possibilities as he wanted, willed, and worked for it to be.

After reading several months of Nate's forward journals, primed I was to reshape my life's focus. Nate's thoughts, coupled with a quote that hit deep in my soul, "Don't let the life you have now distract you from the life you want," positioned me to begin crafting the future I have always desired.

Over the next 52 weeks, I invite you to start the journey to your future with Nate. Each week you will read one of Nate's journal entries. I encourage you to re-read the journal each day of the week and respond to the reflective questions and action steps included for the week.

I refer to the questions and actions steps as the "so what, now what" part of journaling forward. Again, throughout the week, I hope you will write your forward journal entries. I trust you will begin crafting a vision for your own life, a life full of the incredible experiences you want, will, and commit to working on.

Journey Forward:

This is your journey forward, so we want you to use this book in the way that best serves you. Maybe you just want to read this collection of journal entries to be encouraged and allow Nate's words to lend you a spiritual helping hand. We invite you to take advantage of the reflective prompts included after each entry. If that is your choice, let us provide you a road map.

What to Expect:

- 52 Journal Entries (one per week) plus 3 Bonus Entries
- Prompts after each journal encourage you to reflect, write, and act to get to the place you want to go.

What You Need:

- Someplace to capture your thoughts (Nate suggests a laptop; Robin prefers a bound journal with lines and a black ink pen.)

What to Do:

- Get started today!
- Email us at journeyforward@gmail.com to let us know how it's going.

Week 1

Journal Forward

Good day, Journal,

Who could have imagined that 'Journaling Forward' would be ubiquitous in the lives of people across America? When you first started sharing your daily Journal, many people thought it odd to write about experiences you had not yet lived. Others, I am sure, while attempting to spare your feelings, thought you were merely weird.

Why would anyone be so comfortable freely sharing their innermost thoughts and feelings? Who were you is another common question I suspect was being proposed to imagine living the life you want to live in your mind first? Check out this fool Nate Turner, I believe, was a prevailing thought. Who is he to think he has the power to change how he feels each day? Who is he to expect he can control the direction of his life by writing down imagined life experiences as if they are the happenings of the life he lives.

But now, here we are. We, Dr. Wilson, and I published the Journal. Dr. Wilson did the hard part. She asked insightful questions. Dr. Wilson provided context for people to become the best version of themselves when using the Journal. Not only did she do the hard stuff like give readers exercises to discover who they were and who they most wanted to be, but she did so while at the same time making me look good.

Incredibly, Dr. Wilson similarly made me appear genuinely intelligent, convincing the masses to believe reading and listening to me has value. She took the ramblings of a sometimes-admitted crazy man to offer a process of calm and normalcy for those going stir-crazy forced to live through the Coronavirus Pandemic.

When I say admitted, I am not referencing a therapist greeting me with a straight jacket and handcuffs at the entrance of a mental hospital. Relax! I'm fine. Yet, I will never lie or attempt in any way to deny that I experience depression from time to time. Depression is a deadly serious matter, and to be mentally healthy, we must be honest with ourselves and others.

So good or bad, I even journaled about the moments when I was down, way down deep in the dumps. As it turns out, the thing that I first believed would make me appear abnormal, seem too emotionally vulnerable became my calling card.

That's right; the most authentic aspect of the real me made me relatable to the majority. During that time, as I now understand, countless numbers of people were down and out. So many folks were looking for a path to reimagine their reality, hoping to find a way to make enduring the depressing Pandemic palatable.

I used to think it was only a typical expression that there are times when life is analogous to a lightning strike. But I now know first-hand that the words are more than a quaint phrase; the idiom is a profound truth.

Before we started working to turn my journals into a book, a website, an app, lightning struck. The Coronavirus Pandemic hit the world.

Suddenly, people previously able to mask their true feelings with material possession found themselves reduced to covering their noses and mouths with scarves and bandanas. Unexpectedly, folks who ordinarily drowned their sorrows in bars and nightclubs instead could only overdose on bad news and media exploitation. Without warning, segments of society notoriously known for self-medicating with mobile app arranged sexual encounters had to confront the realities of loving only and living solely with oneself.

There was nowhere to go. There was no way to escape the new world. We were all Sheltered in Place, Socially Isolated, and in many cases, quarantined with only me, myself, and I. The only way to get through an unimaginable depressing reality was to do what I had been doing. So I shared journaling forward, a way to imagine living the life you always wanted to live.

And thus, the right time and right place birthed a national movement. Seemingly overnight, 'Journaling Forward' took on greater meaning than just reading the ramblings of a hopeful, sometimes angry, the always crazy Black man.

'Journaling Forward' became a tool to fight the depressive times of the Coronavirus Pandemic. 'Journaling Forward' grew into a self-reflective, totally affordable mental health tool. A cerebral sanity instrument was 'Journaling Forward,' offering anyone an opportunity to honestly ask critically important questions. Such as, "who am I now, and who do I want those who love and care for me to say I was if today was my last day."

'Journaling Forward' first freed me of feelings and thoughts that limited my ability to live my best life. Then journaling did something completely unexpected and so much better than anything I had imagined. 'Journaling Forward' pardoned others from being prisoners of their worst thoughts and feelings. 'Journaling Forward' illustrated for others that they too could be the best versions of themselves and live the life they always imagined.

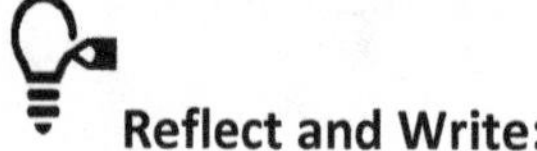

Reflect and Write:

Nate shared with you that 'Journaling Forward' first freed him of feelings and thoughts that limited his ability to live his best life. Take a moment to reflect on today's journal. Then write your responses to the following questions in your own journal.

- So, what is it? What does it, as in what does your best life look like in your mind? Dream audaciously. Free your mind. Write what your best life looks like right now.
- What if any feelings are limiting your ability to live your best life?
- What if anything must change TODAY for you to move towards your best life TOMORROW?
- What is one thing you will do today to take the restraints off and propel yourself towards your best life?

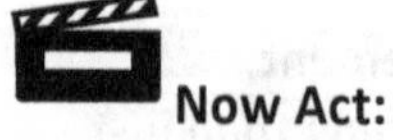

Now Act:

One of the many reasons Nate didn't stop journaling forward was because those of us with who he initially shared the entries looked forward to those entries.

Journey Forward:

Quite honestly, we expected and even demanded that a new entry hit our inbox daily.

While you don't have to do what Nate has done, share your hopes, dreams, and plans with the world, having people to hold you accountable for living your best life does make a world of difference. So, as you begin to chart the path towards the best version of yourself, give some thought to who will be there to hold you accountable? Choose wisely.

Those you select should not be people who regularly dish out false flattery, proclaiming you did something of value when everyone knows you didn't. Nor should the people you choose be skeptics, finding it nearly impossible to say anything positive. To be who you always imagined being, you need people in your life who are optimistic, focused, and straight-shooters. For your accountability partners, you need people who love you for you, who see your enormous potential, and only want what's best for you.

Now identify that person or people. Write him/her/them a letter briefly explaining what you are up to, working to be the best version of you possible, and how he/she/they can help. It might even help if you share this entire journal entry from Nate with them too.

Week 2

Purpose

Good Day, Journal,

On this day, there is no need to be sad or mad. There is absolutely no reason to be disappointed or disgusted. There is no way you can justify being evil or vindictive.

Ups and downs are part of your life. Traversing through mountain tops and valleys is how God designed you. Doing the unthinkable is your middle name. You are a miracle worker. A miracle worker is what you are, and your job, which should come as no surprise to you, is to make miracles happen.

Long ago, you were assigned a mission to do what others would not do. Nobody else received your purpose; it was you who received those instructions on Route 12 and 20. And it is still you who bears the burden of honoring the mission. After all these years, you are still in the miracle-working business.

The ancient writing states that "called are many but chosen are only a few."[i] Many people could be miracle workers. But unlike you, they have chosen to ignore their call, hiding among the frightened and lazy assembly of people who wait on others to perform miracles to make miracles happen for them. You do not sit idly waiting on extraordinary events or others to perform miracles for you; you chose to answer the call; you perform miracles yourself.

I am a miracle worker; I make miracles happen. So, I guess I'll get to work immediately and relentlessly because countless numbers of people are waiting on a phenomenon today.

Your responsibilities as a miracle worker are vast, but so too is your ability. Per the scripture, "to whom much is given is much required[ii]." You were gifted miraculous power; thus, you must provide miracles for others.

Your gifts are both divine and eternal. Where others see and smell shit, you see and smell sugar. Shit is the manure that fertilizes all vegetation, including sugar cane. Without shit, there would be no sugar cane. Absent shit sugar would not taste as sweet, and the things baked with sugar would not smell as sweet. I guess you could say that you turn shit into sugar.

While others whine about their condition, you understand that anything worth having comes with challenges and likely includes tears. When folks say that "the best is yet to come," rarely do we acknowledge that the best almost always comes for us when we are willing to go through challenges. Success can not be separated from those difficulties that often bring us to our knees and cause us to shed many tears.

In this life, the more complex the challenge, the more significant the outcome. The more bodacious the dream, the more likely there will be tears, buckets of tears. And so there it is again, evidence of the manifestation of being a miracle worker. While others whine about the challenges, fearing tears, you cry tears of joy.

You understand what others fail to appreciate; tears are the moisturizer for your dreams. Without tears, our dreams have no chance of being transported into the reality of our mind springing us forward to our best life. I suppose it would not be an exaggeration to say that you turn whine into spring water. Your life flows along consistently thanks in considerable measure because of the water released from your eyes.

But perhaps the most significant responsibility you have as a miracle worker is helping those without vision avoid doing things that will lead to their demise. You are the humane aid like a white cane or a seeing-eye dog, helping the blind see.

Helping those without vision see their way forward is not easy, especially when the prescription for sight is for those who do not have literal blindness. Daily, your call is to support and assist those whose blindness extends far beyond the loss of eyesight.

You must help those whose eyesight is 20/20 see – to see that there is a better way to educate the underserved masses, to see that there is a better way to build communities for the masses of disenfranchised, marginalized groups, to envision the way to eradicating the parenting policies which often lead to

National social-economic decline, and to see in many cases for the first time that there is another way, a better way to be human.

Your life is miraculous! You are a miracle-worker! Now live out your purpose. Deliver miracles today!

Reflect and Write:

Like Nate, you, too, are a miracle worker. Created are we all for a divine purpose and mission. Take a moment to reflect on today's journal. Then write your responses to the following questions in your own journal.

"Nobody else received your purpose."

- What is your purpose? Seriously, what is the ONE thing that no one else can do but you?
- Who in your life/your community/your world needs you to fulfill your purpose?
- What barriers have you encountered on the path towards your purpose?
- Now that you have identified the barriers, push them aside. What will you do TODAY to make progress in your purpose?

Now Act:

Decide on three things you will do this week that moves you towards fulfilling your purpose. No step is too small. Write them down and revisit this list six days from now. Then, be sure to share them with your accountability person.

You do have at least one person to hold you accountable for fulfilling your purpose, right? Did you complete last week's task?

Journey Forward:

Week 3

Courage

Good Day, Journal,

Today, I've decided to live to my potential. For just one day and one day only, I am making a deal with myself to live up to my ability. On this day, I've decided not to slack, not to make any excuses but instead to do everything to my maximum capability.

Of course, I should make this agreement with myself daily. I should live up to my potential every day without exception. And I will.

I will agree daily to keep all excuses out of my mouth. I promise that I'll give my all to avoid behavior that causes me to slack off from giving my best effort so that I might live my best life. Instead, I will live a life committed to habits and a routine that makes it possible for me to live up to my unlimited God-given ability.

No matter what I commit to throughout my life, regardless of how long I give myself permission to be great, which by the way, is the full extent of my life, the first mandatory decision each day is to live today to its maximum. I will ride or die with today, and in so doing, tomorrow will ride or die with me.

Everything I want to be in the future rides on what I do today. Everyone I want to love me in the future counts on how I love them today. Every dollar I anticipate earning, each award I envision winning, all the books I expect to sell, and every single solitary speaking venue I imagine talking in all depend on the relationship I have with today.

How I treat today epitomizes how I treat anything, how I treat everything. What I do today illustrates what I'm willing to do every day.

There is no tomorrow without today. There can be no brighter day without living up to my potential right now. There is no need to hope for tomorrow if I am unwilling to bust my ass being the best version of myself possible at this very moment.

I will ride or die with today so that tomorrow will ride or die with me. A such today, I commit to being great.

Today, I will do all that is in my ability to make my dream life a reality. Today, I will inspire others by how I live my life that all who know and meet me might strive to be the best versions of themselves possible.

I have the courage today to do what I feared doing yesterday. Today, I live in harmony with tomorrow. I will ride or die with today, so that should the Universe gift me another day to be better than any day previously, tomorrow will ride or die with me.

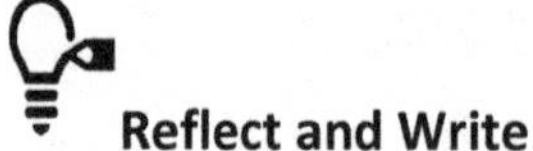

Reflect and Write:

Choosing to avoid excuses takes courage. It's your turn to do today what you feared doing yesterday. Take a moment to reflect on today's journal. Then write your responses to the following questions in your own journal.

- What would it look like if you did not make any excuses today and instead did everything to your maximum capability?
- What are two new habits you need to develop to live this life to your most complete ability?
- How will you treat today so that it is different than yesterday?

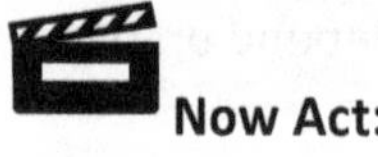

Now Act:

"How I treat today epitomizes how I treat anything, how I treat everything. What I do today illustrates what I'm willing to do every day."

Journey Forward:

Decide for each day this week. Be specific. Commit to making each day better than the day before. Revisit your journal entries each day to keep yourself accountable.

Week 4

Dream

Good Day, Journal,

Today is a big day, a huge day. I dare say one of the most meaningful days in your entire life. On this day, everything about your future hinges. What you do today propels or plummets your legacy. So without question, today matters.

Are you ready for this day? Eighty thousand-plus people packed into the Mercedes Benz Stadium in Atlanta, Georgia, to hear you speak. Say that one more time with emphasis while smacking yourself upside the head. Eighty thousand-plus people packed into the Mercedes Benz Stadium in Atlanta, Georgia, to hear you speak.

Today's the day where one of the things you have always envisioned will soon be a reality. Shortly, you will have the opportunity to share the words of wisdom God gave you to impart to the lives of others.

We all have the potential to be a vessel of knowledge to bring the good news, so don't take this opportunity for granted. Remember, you are replaceable instantly; someone is willing to supplant you in the twinkling of an eye.

What are you going to share? It would be best if you gave them something they never heard before. Offer something easy to remember, something that will resonate for days, weeks, months, and potentially years to come. The clock is ticking. It will be show time real soon.

"Time to Leave the Bunny Hills." I think that's what I'm going to name my speech. "Time to Leave the Bunny Hills." I will share a childhood experience of learning to ski with the audience, including how the only hills I ever skied were the bunny hills.

The bunny hills represent the no effort aspects of our lives. We can walk to the top of the bunny hill with little effort and, more importantly, without taking hardly any risk, we can journey down the bunny hill. The ski slope bunny hill is so effortless and of little danger that even the youngest children hate being on the bunny hill.

But figuratively, bunny hills are where we find most adults in life — doing the same old easy repetitive actions that neither challenge us coming or going. Up each morning and in bed each night, knowing full well that the life we live is far less than we desire and are capable of living. And despite having a clear and present view of far more significant opportunities, as the progressively higher hills are lined up in order of difficulty next to the bunny hill, we choose to stay on the bunny hill. We elect to remain in an unchallenged, unfulfilling, undesired life.

Get off the bunny hill is what I'm going to say. To get the most out of this life, your only life, to see things you never saw, to do stuff you only dreamed of doing, you are going to have to leave the bunny hill. To live your best life, to master yourself, the slopes of an authentic life demand that you must leave the bunny hill.

I left the bunny hill some years ago. I could not continue walking up and sliding down the same financial advisory slope any longer. In its place, I saw the glorious hills of writing and speaking. I envisioned the rewards of sharing things that could change lives with the masses– tips so simple that anyone could live their best life.

Today, I am healthier, wealthier, and wiser than I ever imagined. I am so because I decided to stay off the bunny hill.

I hope the roof is open when I speak today. I want the audience to see what I see in my mind's eye daily. The glorious sun shining down on me reminds me that today is a great day. If I continue to stay off the bunny hills, my future is brighter than ever.

Until tomorrow,

Nate

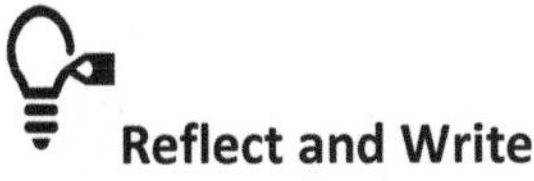

Reflect and Write:

Nothing changes without action. Take a moment to reflect on today's journal. Then write your responses to the following questions in your own journal.

- List one aspect of your legacy. Think BIG. DREAM.
- What will you do within the next hour that propels your legacy? What will you have done by the time you go to bed tonight to move your desired future forward?
- What is your current "Bunny Hill"?
- List 3 action steps you need to move you off this bunny hill onto a progressively higher elevation.
- Reflect on your responses. Write a journal entry aimed at what life will be like due to the changes listed above.

Now Act:

Each entry from Nate provides a glimpse into the life he envisioned for himself and those he loves. What do you envision for your future? Seriously. What story do you want others to talk about in your life? Write it down.

Record what you want now. Scripture tells us, "Write the vision and make it plain on tablets..." So, get to writing.

Week 5

Aim

Good day, Journal,

Everyone says that they want to be rich. Lots of folks claim they want to be famous. Rich and famous are all too familiar words repeated by people everywhere. The truth, however, is that wanting to be rich and famous has little to do with being rich and famous.

To be rich and famous, you must sacrifice, fail, grow from the sacrifice and failure, keep moving forward, and start again. There are no shortcuts to being rich and famous. Rejection is not optional. Failure is not discretionary. Rejection and failure are mandatory.

When I was a child, all I thought about was being rich and famous. I wanted only to be a professional basketball player. Yet, no matter how much I claimed to want to play professionally, the truth is that I wasn't willing to do what was necessary to be a professional basketball player. Namely, I wasn't interested in the sacrifice and failure required to be rich and famous. Not to mention, I was only 5'10.5".

My height, while a limitation, was not a deterrent, but my mind was a significant impediment, so I never became a professional basketball player. Full disclosure, I never became many of the things I said I wanted to be for the very same reason – my betraying mind.

Back in the day, I was not interested in sacrificing, failing, growing from the sacrifice and failure, and doing those things over and over and repeatedly. I didn't know what was inside me earlier in life, namely that the space between my two ears mattered way more than anything outside of me. It wasn't so long ago that my mind played tricks on me.

Today, I get it completely. These days I not only understand, but I embrace this process of becoming rich and famous. First, you must sacrifice, fail, grow from the sacrifice and failure. Then you must keep moving forward and start the sacrifice, fail, and grow process all over again and again.

Fortunately, today, I am no longer motivated by fame. I'm not even driven by wealth. As I now know, fame and wealth are outcomes. My mind no longer plays tricks on me.

If all you are interested in are the outcomes, what will you do once you reach the destination? The answer is simple. Most people quit when they get the desired result because that's all they planned.

Thank goodness I stopped concerning myself with the results of being rich and famous because when I did, everything changed. My place on the planet changed because I changed how I processed and thought about being rich and famous.

The day I started channeling all my time and energy to the process of being the best version of me possible each day, my life took off. No longer weighed down by trying to become rich and famous, I became rich and famous. No longer obsessed with proving to others that I would be rich and famous, I started living the life I always imagined.

On this day, I will not chase being rich or famous. I will all the remaining days of my life merely concentrate on finding the best way, the most natural way, the authentic way to experience a joyful life. Today, I gladly embrace my responsibility to help, serve, and make sure others know their life matters free of any desire or expectation of fame and fortune.

I do not live to be rich and famous. Which does not mean I lack gratitude for being in excellent health, possessing abundant wealth, or the ability to share timeless wisdom. On the contrary, I am so very appreciative of the remarkable life the Universe allows me to live each day.

Yet now that my mind no longer plays tricks on me, I understand the truth about being rich and famous. Both are overrated; society misconstrues both. I know several broken, rich, and famous people, society's upper crest existing poor in spirit and infamous, defamed in character so many despite their wealth and privilege.

Journey Forward:

As long as I have breath, my aim will be unchanged. Today, I understand my life mission clearly. My call is to be the best version of myself possible, to make my family and loved ones proud, and to do my part to leave the planet better when I leave it than it was when I arrived. If that makes me rich and famous, so be it.

Reflect and Write:

I recently read the following about aim, "Our brain is constantly at work prioritizing tasks and goals. Do you know what priority your brain uses when it makes decisions on how to invest your time? Most of us don't because we haven't articulated our priorities." Take a moment to reflect on today's journal. Then write your responses to the following questions in your own journal.

- What is the aim of your life? Write it here.
- What limitations have you placed on your mind that work to convince you that achieving your aim is impossible? List them all, yes, all of them, here!
- Are your current actions moving you towards your aim, or are they sabotaging your quest towards the best version of you? If you are self-sabotaging, what must you do differently to immediately place yourself on the path towards fulfilling your life's aim?

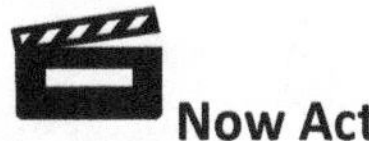

Now Act:

What will you concentrate on today/this week that will propel you towards fulfilling your life's aim?

Share your aim with your accountability partner.

Write the following questions on post-it notes and place them in prominent places you frequent throughout your day: bathroom mirror, refrigerator, car dashboard, office wall.

1. Is what I am about to do going to move me closer to my aim?
2. If not, why would I do it?

Week 6

Time

Good day, Journal,

What else should we talk about at 3:46 am other than the time? Yes, we're talking about time. Not the band, not the musical group that featured Morris Day, Jerome Benton, Alexander O'Neal, Jimmy Jam, and Terry Lewis. No, we're talking about the 'time,' the aspect of life that keeps getting away from us.

Time as in the seasons that fly by amazingly fast because we were having so much fun. 'Time' is that elusive race against which we all lose. Yes, that time, those gifted moments made available by the Universe to live our best life, the time that waits for no one. Yes, that same time when annually we reflect on the past 365 days and sing ♪ For auld Lang syne, my dear, For auld Lang syne, ♪.[iii] Yes, we're talking about time.

Growing up, I wish I knew as much about time or cared about time half as much as I cared about Morris Day and 'The Time.' I remember wanting to prove the validity of Morris Day's words, "gigolos get lonely too."[iv] I wanted everyone to know I was ♪C-O-O-L♪.[v]

From my' walk,' the Zoot Suits, the dance moves, and of course, women, I wanted to be Morris Day so bad. During my high school senior year, I placed a sign on my locker that read "Nate AKA Morris Day." If I could have, I would have changed my phone number to '777-9311.'

It's painfully incongruous and embarrassingly ironic to note now that my favorite group did not inspire me to use my time wisely. Instead, 'The Time' only encouraged me to waste time. Failing to appreciate time must have been what my elders were attempting to warn me about when I fell in love with 'Ice cream castles in the summertime.'

No doubt, my obsession with 'The Time' rather than time epitomizes the meaning of George Bernard Shaw's words, "youth is wasted on the young."

When I was young, I wasted my youth being 'wild and loose,' hoping to 'get it up,' getting ready to have a real good time, and crying over the 'girl' who went away.

In those "good old days," I did all the things that would not serve me well in the future. As a young man trying to mimic Morris Day, I watched carelessly as my youth took flight and flew far, far away.

Today, according to the chronology of my life, I am now a middle-aged man. Supposedly, I am on the downside of life. Purportedly, I have used up more than half of my time. If this is true, I must admit it. I wish I had more time.

Yes, we are talking about the time I wasted that I would love to retrieve, the time I desperately want to reclaim to now use wisely. But alas, there is no recovering or retrieving any bygone time. Once 'time' is gone, it's gone for good!

Life's time allocation is nothing like a political blowhard incessantly pontificating, demanding more time whenever another political blowhard interjects during their grandstanding. No, in real life, living outside of partisan politics, once any grain of sand drops from the top of the hourglass to the bottom, the sand remains forever at the bottom. You can't rewind time, nor can you undo wasted moments.

There are no Disney or Pixar animated miracles when the sand falls from the top. The sands of time do not wondrously float back to the top. Once the grains reach the floor of the hourglass, they stick to the bottom for eternity. And as each grain of sand represents so eloquently, once the moment passes, it is gone forever.

You can wish for more time in this life, but your petition for more time is like a bell ringing at the end of school, dismissing. You get what time the Universe gifts; nobody, not even you, shall receive more time.

I suppose this is why I wake up often in the wee hours of the morning. I presume, therefore, that explains why my brain routinely feels like an automobile motor pushed during an Indy car race – overheated and worn down.

I now know what I had no concept of when I sang along with 'The Time.' Life is not a song to sing with 'The Time'; life is a race against time.

Journey Forward:

Sooner than later, we all run out of time. But before I do, while I yet have time today, I'm going to accomplish as much as possible. Today, I'm going to be as kind and loving as I can. On this day, I'm going to work like hell to let the world know that I was here and that I did some good with my time.

What time is it? It's time to help, serve, and make sure others know their life matters? What time is it? It's time to work on remaining in excellent health, holding on to abundant wealth, and sharing timeless wisdom. What time is it? It's time to use whatever time that remains, living life as I always imagined.

Reflect and Write:

I suspect you are like Nate and can recount lots of time that you have lost. I am sure there are countless minutes you have spent on things and people that have yielded no fruit. The reality is, as Nate wrote, "you get what time the Universe gifts; nobody, not even you, shall receive more time."

However, all hope is not lost. The Universe has gifted you with today. And if you're fortunate, there are minutes, hours, days, months, even years remaining in your life. So, the ball is in your court. How will you make the most of your time?

Take a minute to reflect on these time-based questions below. You are worth all the time you will invest.

- Go ahead and lament. Take a moment to write down your biggest regret as it relates to time. Then, get it out of your head so you can move forward.

- You have somewhere around 168 hours available to you this week, depending on the day and time you read this. So, to end the week feeling like you have moved closer to the life you want, think about how you will allocate those hours.

- Identify your most significant time wasters. Write them down. Which of them will you commit to eliminating this week?

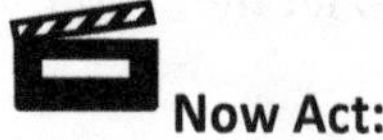

Now Act:

Please take a moment to note. This is week 6 of your journey to living out your destiny to be your best self. As you are six weeks into your expedition, you should have at least one person holding you accountable by now.

You have tried your hand at creating a week's worth of action steps to move forward. And you have written the vision for life as you know it will be.

It's time (pun intended) to purge. What must you eliminate to move this journey forward? For some, it will be discontinuing mindless TV watching. For others, you will cease spending countless hours on social media. All of us must do some analysis, including a potential reallocation of how we spend our time.

What must you eliminate (or at least drastically reduce) to reclaim time to get to the life you desire? Write it down. Tell your accountability partner. Ask them to text you a daily check-in to see how you're doing at no longer wasting time.

Journey Forward:

Week 7

Love

Good day, Journal,

"I love me some me." I know that when I say that I love myself out loud that way, it might come off as arrogant, narcissistic, and maybe even slightly ludicrous, but I do not intend to do so. I say, "I love me some me" because loving oneself is the most important thing any of us can and need to do. Because if anyone is ever going to love anyone else correctly, we must completely love ourselves first.

People often confound me. Daily we profess to love others. But when you look at us, when you speak with us, when you spend any amount of time with us, one can tell almost immediately that we don't know what love is, much less love ourselves.

Our appearance, while having no physical debility, more often than not, is less than optimal. Despite knowing that we are not taking care of the Temple appropriately, we continue each day doing those things that cause the Temple to crack in an ill-advised way. We sit and watch the Temple crumble and fall apart unnecessarily fast.

Intentionally and consciously, we do things that potentially shorten our life span—daily living a life that fails to exhibit the devotion one should have for oneself. We regularly demonstrate why and how not to love us, particularly revealing to those we would most like to love us. From the earliest introduction to our outward appearance, we deliberately and willfully infer first and foremost for all to see that we don't like much less love ourselves.

Each day, there are those of us whose spoken words are unloving. There is no way that we could believe for a second that we love ourselves, given the harsh, evil-spirited words we speak into existence. "I can't," "someone is better than me," "they're smarter than me," "I'll try," or "I don't have that gift" are a few of the more polite less than loving examples of the words that we allow to spring forth out of our mouths daily.

We speak out loud for others to hear that we do not love ourselves. Yet, somehow foolishly, we expect that others must love us. Irrationally, we insist that others should trust us to love them.

So, I remind myself daily, and I say it out loud frequently, "I love me some me" because I know loving me is key to loving others. Should my outside appearance not provide some tangible inference that I love me, I know visual-leaning humans will easily reject me as one worthy of love. Dismiss me they surely will as one capable of loving others in great mass.

Moreover, if the words that come out of my mouth do not initially convey the loving thoughts that need to exist in my mind first, all hope is lost. As I speak, so am I. "I love me some me" because I desire to live up to the directive for being a model of the Universe's love.

The ancient scripture that provides the foundation for my life includes two directives that I contemplate daily. The first is "Thou shalt love the Lord thy God with all thy heart, and with all thy soul, and with all thy mind."[vi] And the second is "Thou shalt love thy neighbor as thyself."[vii]

Whether one recognizes a greater power than them as the Lord, God, Spirit, Universe, or whatever is up to them. However, what's unquestionably clear is that a Life Source exists, making it possible, allowing each of us to see a new day.

It is irrefutable that humans are not the most powerful, knowing presence on the planet. Thank God for that, for if we were the omnipotent, omnipresent beings, this planet would have ceased to exist long ago. We are much too messy to be all-powerful!

So then, what does the first directive require that I do each day? The first directive expects me to be in love with, to adore completely, to show through each beat of my heart, via the absolute essence of the spirituality of my soul, and with all the intellectual thoughts of my mind that I recognize I have control of only one thing – the way I express and share 'love' with the Universe.

I am a caretaker; we are all caretakers of the planet. We all share the same responsibility to love all living things that contain the All Mighty' s presence. We are all actors receiving the same universal direction to "be love" with all our hearts, souls, and minds.

And the second mandate is similar in importance and urgency to the first: the requirement to love our neighbors as ourselves. So daily, we need to ask ourselves, "Can one love a neighbor when one does not love themselves?" "What definition of love should a neighbor ascribe to those of us who, by outward appearance and inward beliefs that manifest in conversation, clearly show that we do not love ourselves?"

So, "I love me some me." "I love me some me" because loving me is a requirement to fulfill my call; it is essential to become the best version of myself possible. 'Loving me some me' is a requirement for helping, serving, and making sure others know that life matters that they are loved. "Loving me some me" is justified and demanded by the Creator, the Author of Love.

Reflect and Write:

If you began reading this journal the first week of the year, you picked up this week's entry in mid-February, the month the world declares as love month. So, let's go with it and make this "I love me some me" month.

Take a minute to reflect on the questions below. Show yourself some love!

- In this week's journal, Nate wrote, "I remind myself daily, and I say it out loud frequently, "I love me some me" because I know loving me is key to loving others." So stop what you are doing, walk to the mirror and say, "I love you." How did it feel?
- Let's stick with this self-love idea for just a minute. Please make a list of 5 reasons you love yourself.
- How was that? Was it a challenge? What is getting in the way of you loving you?

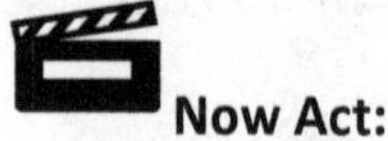

Now Act:

Write yourself a love note. But write it to the person you will be this time next year. What accomplishments will you be celebrating? What milestones will you have hit?

Now place the letter in a sealed, self-addressed, stamped envelope. Give it to your accountability person. Assign them the task of setting a reminder on their phone to drop the letter in the mail to you precisely 50 weeks from today. What will the current you be glad to celebrate with next year's you?

Week 8

Today

Good day, Journal,

No one will outwork me. Today there will not be a person on the face of the Earth that will be able to claim they outperformed me. For anyone to declare they outworked me would be a bald-faced lie. A slim few people on the planet may work as hard, but no one will defeat me today.

Outworking me cannot happen. I must not be defeated today. My entire future depends on having a laser focus and expending a relentless effort today. The life that I always imagined is waiting on the other side of not being outworked.

Being outworked today is, at best, an imagined life deal breaker. Failing to rise to the occasion, which is to neglect the Universe's presenting of the gift called today, giving anything less than my maximum effort is non-negotiable. To be the best version of me requires that I honor the Universe's bounty and forbid anyone to outwork me.

I cannot; I must not allow anyone to outwork me. I have got to put in work for real; I got to do real work today. Seriously, I have no time to play 'work' today. I can't be working for play. The work I do must result in pay.

Nor shall I make any allowances for busy work either. No shuffling papers from one side of the desk to the other. No doing the easy stuff first, things that are on my unspoken but genuine 'comfortable list.' No acting as if the difficult and uncomfortable things do not demand my full and undivided attention all day long.

Today, you will not find me pretending that somehow if I do the easy stuff first, the hard things will magically take care of themselves. That's called denial, and denial is not a river in Egypt.

Denial makes you delusional. Denial and delusion be damned today. Hear this and hear this loud and clear, "if you don't do the work, the work will undo you." "If you deny the required work exists, the life you desire will deny you exist."

The life you always imagined is embedded deep inside the complex tasks and the uncomfortable action items. So, do not delay putting in work because you are just putting off the inevitable. To reach your potential, you must press forward and stop procrastinating. You must get to work; no one must be able to outwork you today. You must do the work or watch in horror as the work undoes you, as the life you desire denies you exist.

Each day, millions of people, just like you, proclaim that they want to live the life they always imagined. The masses claim that they want to be the best version of themselves, yet most never scratch the surface of their potential. Wanting to live your best life is easy, but working to live your best life is an entirely different story. Being your best, living the life you always imagined is hard; doing what is necessary is damn hard.

Today do not be who you were yesterday; do not be who millions will be today. Today, be the one person the Universe can count on to outwork everyone. Be the person who used every second of the gift of today, the one person who allocated all their time and energy to lay the groundwork to live their best life.

Outwork them all today. Outwork everyone today. Do not let your mind wander on things you have no control. Do not suffer the constant distraction of fools.

Focus squarely on your envisioned life. Then, with your mind's eye, see all the hope and possibility of that life, your best life experiences. And anytime during the day, should you lose focus or get distracted, take a deep breath, refocus, and concentrate once more on being the best version of yourself again.

Today, I will outwork everyone. Today, no one will lay claim to having outperformed me. I will first beat others in my mind. Later, I will outwork everyone with the thoughts in my heart. I will use the powerful emotive images and the force of the Universe to keep me focused intently and working relentlessly to live the life I have always imagined.

Today, no one can, and no one will outwork me. On this day, I will not be defeated.

Journey Forward:

Reflect and Write:

As I read this journal for probably the 10th time, several statements stuck out to me. Those statements are listed below. Take some time this week to reflect on each of them. Next, respond to the questions that follow. Then get to work!

- "My entire future depends on having a laser focus and expending a relentless effort today. The life that I always imagined is waiting on the other side of not being outworked." So what will I expend all of my effort on today? This week?

- "The life you always imagined is embedded deep inside the difficult tasks and the uncomfortable action items." Hence what complex tasks lie ahead? List them here.

- "Be the person who used every second of the gift of today, the one person who allocated all their time and energy to lay the groundwork to live their best life." What groundwork will you lay this week?

Now Act:

It's been two months. We want to hear from you. Send us an e-mail at journeyforward@gmail.com to let us know how it's going.

Week 9

Give

Good Day, Journal,

Today, we are going to do something long overdue. Today, we will show the world that the idiom "beggars can't be choosers" is dead wrong.

From this day forward, the entire team and I will spend no fewer than one day per week helping, serving, and showing others that their life matters. Thus, for the totality of at least one day, 24 consecutive hours, we shall spend no less than ten percent of our weekly time, talent, and profits helping, serving, and making sure the "so-called beggars" know their lives matter.

We should give all of ourselves to those in the greatest need, just as we would do for ourselves if those who have the greatest need were us. Why? Because there should be no question about how each of us loves ourselves. Perhaps then, if we looked at the oppressed and disenfranchised as if they were us, we would reconsider our charitable efforts and rethink our beliefs about "beggars and choosers."

Only when you experience your humanity inwardly are you able to express humanity outwardly. It's nearly impossible to give others what you are, not yourself. When you lack humanity, you cannot provide humanity. As such, the existence and measure of one's humanity manifest itself in the lives of others, most notably in the way we treat "the least of them."

How humane are we? How much humanity is inside us? It's time; the time is now for us to look deep down inside our minds and search the depths of our hearts for more humanity. It's time that we live up to the teachings "love thy neighbor as thyself."

And while the historically marginalized and geographically underserved rarely, if ever, live next to us, they are neighbors on planet earth. Therefore, it is past time that we demonstrated in word and deed "loving our neighbors as ourselves" and discontinued propagating the asinine expression "beggars can't be choosers."

Today, we'll show the world. If anyone deserves a choice, if anybody ought to have a say, it is those who seemingly never have a choice; it's the insultingly labeled "beggars." If only for one day a week, today we will give the "have nots" an opportunity to choose a day without bag lunches, hand me down clothing, shaking cups, wearing "please help me..." signs, birdbaths, or sleeping on a cot in a shelter. Today, we're going to treat the inappropriately described "beggars" like ourselves.

Today, we're offering the disenfranchised an enormous buffet, a spread of food the likes that many have never seen, that they may choose to eat whatever and how much they like. After the meal fit for royalty, we're taking our fellow brothers and sisters on a shopping spree so that they might choose whatever they want to wear.

It will be a clothing extravaganza. A chance to pick and choose brand new stuff. An opportunity to not settle for items offered from the bin of used garments. Instead, they will take with them fresh fashions only, not outfits privileged people no longer desire to wear.

Finally, we're going to offer the option of checking into several of the city's best hotels. They can choose to enjoy the luxurious creature comforts we all so easily take for granted. Opulent showers, baths, fluffy towels and robes, designer sheets, plush pillows and mattresses, picturesque views of the city, and room service will be just the minimum offered to everyone.

To be clear, I know this is not the solution to the causes of homelessness. Resolving homelessness requires structural and systemic changes to our economy, healthcare system, educational institutions, and the like. As needed to address nearly all other societal ills, eradicating homelessness calls for a massive precise reconstructive surgery on this Nation's heart. But because we understand the magnitude of the problem coupled with the realization that tomorrow offers no promises and that our daily call is to be better today than yesterday, today we are going to do the best we can do to help, serve, and make sure others know their life matters.

Today is not about individual supreme health, abundant personal wealth, or respected timeless wisdom. On this day, we will show the world that the idiom "beggars can't be choosers" is not wrong. Moreover, we'll show that if anyone deserves to choose, those resigned to live each day without choice are the most deserving. Today is a personal accounting and a universal assessment of our humanity.

Reflect and Write:

"It's time; the time is now for us to look deep down inside our minds and search the depths of our hearts for more humanity. It's time that we live up to the teachings "love thy neighbor as thyself."

By now, you have read enough journals to have fallen in love with yourself. Equipped, you are for the next step, which is to love thy neighbor as thyself. If you don't love yourself, you cannot love others.

But as was pointed out in the entry, your neighbor is not defined by proximity. Today's journal is about a greater calling to extend love to those who deserve love but rarely receive it.

Take a moment to reflect on the condition of your community. Where is there a need? How might you meet that need?

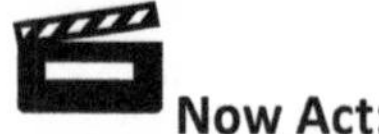

Now Act:

Today's task is to give. Identify an organization that serves the disenfranchised, marginalized, and under-resourced in your community. Then serve. Do not just give money but meet the people where they are. Put faces to the unfortunate statistics and remind the people you meet that their lives matter.

Week 10

Be Relentless

Good day, Journal,

Gatorade asks the question, "is it in you?" Yeah, I know. What do they want to discover that's in or not in you?

Are they asking if the so-called rehydration drink with toxic coloring and artificial sweetener is in you? Or are they seeking an answer to a question you demand a response of yourself daily?

Is it in you today? Is greatness in you today? Is the fire for your best life burning red hot inside you today? Is the relentless determination to help, serve, and make sure others know that their lives matter inside you today? Is the best version of you possible – the 178-pound man of twisted steel with young Denzel sex appeal with abundant wealth and timeless wisdom – living inside in you?

Daily, you must make sure that the best you exist in the flesh and that the best you remain available ready to leap on to the canvas called life eagerly. There's no sense in letting anything good just sit inside you when the world desperately needs you to make it manifest on the outside. Living any day without purpose and passion is like paints and brushes forcibly locked up when an enormous, pristine canvas awaits your artistry.

The best of you matters. The best of you matters a whole lot. And keeping the best you locked up inside not only does not help you, but it also cheats the world; it gravely disappoints the Universe.

That which is inside you did not originate with you. You are not the author or the architect of the inner workings of your being. What's inside you mainly, the good to crucial parts of you are on loan for only a short time. Yet, the bequeath of an extension of life's credit is most likely when you daily share those good things inside you with others.

So, today when it comes to sharing the best of yourself with others, abide by the premise 'the more, the merrier.' Share and share some more, especially if you desire another day. Sharing is not optional whenever you seek another extension of life's credit to be better tomorrow than you will be today.

Is it in you? What's in you is perhaps the best place to start?

Is that championship mettle that life requires to run through walls of disappointment and leap over endless obstacles in you this morning? Is that superhero quality that believes in the best of humanity and that would willingly lay down his life for the wellbeing of the greater good drifting inside you right now? Does that Wiley Coyote relentless spirit of continuing to get up after anvils of hatred and bombs of naysaying attempt to thwart your pursuit of excellence live in you today?

'It' better be in you today! On this day, you may need to bring everything you have available to the party called living the life you always imagined. You will probably need to carry the kitchen sink with you too.

Don't you dare leave anything out of your internal toolbox today! You better make sure you are carrying around and have easy access to all the best stuff you have inside you. Are you ready to give the world the best of you that is available today?

Front and center bring forth the best things you can offer the world. You must not hide the best parts of you today; make sure the best of you is both seen and heard.

Do not shrink today. You dare not forget your God-given responsibility to leave the planet better than it was when you depart than when you arrived.

Is it in you? I believe that it is. I know that it is. Now it's up to you to decide if you will bring the best of you to the forefront today. Right now, you must prove that what's in you is much more than a lot of hot air and BS.

Oh yeah, it's in me! Greatness dwells in me. The relentless pursuit of my best life, a quest I will take up to the end of my days by any means necessary, is in me.

Journey Forward:

Please pay close attention, world. Today you will see what's in me. I'll leave no doubt about how the Universe made me. Get your paper and pencils out, say action, roll the camera; get your popcorn ready.

Today, the entire world will be living witnesses to the solution for the day's question, an eternal matter for our lifetime. Is it in me? Answer: Hell yeah!

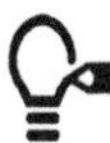

Reflect and Write:

Throughout this week's journal, Nate asked you several questions. Let's revisit a few of those here:

- Is the relentless determination to help, serve, and make sure others know that their lives matter inside you today?

- Is that championship mettle that life requires to run through walls of disappointment and leap over endless obstacles in you this morning?

- Are you ready to give the world the best of you that is available today?

If you answered "Hell NO" to any of these questions, take a moment to adjust your attitude. Start by giving thanks for the mere fact that you were able to read these words today. Then do a quick self-exam. What are three of the best parts of you? Write them down. Say them out loud.

Now, re-read the questions.

Assuredly, you have changed your response to "Hell Yeah" and are ready to move forward with the relentless drive to give the world the best version of you.

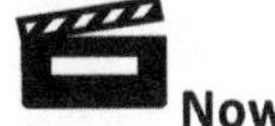

Now Act:

So, today when it comes to sharing the best of yourself with others, abide by the premise 'the more, the merrier.' Share and share some more, especially if you desire another day. Sharing is not optional whenever you seek another extension of life's credit to be better tomorrow than you will be today.

Look back at the list of three of the best parts of you listed above. Who will you share those with today? How will you share it? Be specific. Then do it!

After you have shared, come back here, and let the journal know how it went. What surprised you? What more can you give and how?

Week 11

Time to Remember.

Good day, Journal,

Wow! What a life! As I look back down memory lane, I can hardly believe just how far I've come. I mean, I unquestionably know that I'm here. I don't need anyone to pinch me to make sure that this is real that I'm not dreaming.

Being in excellent health, acquiring abundant wealth, and possessing timeless wisdom is precisely how I always imagined living. Living in this beach house paid for in cash and walking the shoreline every morning is as I accurately envisioned, as evidenced by my 2019 vision board.

What I meant to say was that my journey has been incredible. A trek that, when I look back at it now sometimes, seems all so improbable. While undoubtedly unlikely, it was never impossible. Living my best life was always necessary.

I know only through the grace and mercy of the Creator that any of this is possible. I know that absent the gifted talents of each specially curated spiritual donation, I am nothing. I am no one.

The book and speaking awards on my mantle, the humanitarian plaques on the wall, the service commendations from public officials, the plethora of honorary doctorate degrees I've received for speeches given all over the world seem all so unlikely for someone like me. As a man who considers himself little more than just a guy, what a delightful surprise to find out I can be just a little bit more than I thought. And to think it all started with a walk to the mailbox.

Yeah, I wrote my son because I loved him and didn't want to screw him up or our relationship like my father had done, he and I. I wrote my son on a single postcard, a few words, and instantaneously realized that there wasn't nearly enough space to tell him how much he meant to me.

I wrote my son on a lonely Hallmark greeting card. I used every inch of the available space to discover that the card's true meaning was not the prepopulated sentiment. I found out I needed more space to share lessons about life with my son.

And that lousy written book, yeah, my writing then was nothing like the prose I share with the world today. I got to keep it honest. When I look back on that book, I was not a good writer at all.

But writing my son personalized letters was not intended to be an exhibition of excellent writing. The letters weren't supposed to be available for anyone but him. Yet writing him and then electing to share the messages with others brought out a forgotten, buried part.

I forget how much I loved to write. I forgot about the creative, imaginative stories I wrote as a child. I forgot about the way I wrote in college. I disregarded how I challenged professors every chance I had to see the world to envision the subject matter from my perspective, from another standpoint like that of people like me.

Shamefully, I let my life take over, and I stopped doing the things the Creator embedded inside me. My gifts, the presents that the Universe only offered to me, lay resting in my mind and soul, collecting dust.

I'd not only been wasting my gifts; I was wasting my time on the planet. I was losing my life. Perhaps worst of all, I was also depriving the world of the gifts the Spirit gave me to pay forward and share with others.

For what is a gift, if one withdraws it if one hoards it? Can a gift of a pair of shoes help one who has no footgear if the gift giver keeps the footwear in a gift box in their home where there are numerous pairs of shoes already?

I was the guy with multiple pairs of shoes. I had ideas for helping, serving, and making sure others know their lives matter, but like the guy with lots of shoes packed away, hoarded in his closet, I did not gift the shoes to those who were shoeless.

I left my gifts wrapped up, collecting dust, rotting away in the 'Lost and Found' closet of life. Not only were skeletons in my closet, so too were all the gifts I had to offer the world. Not only were my skills getting dusty on the inside of life's proverbial armoire, but I was also literally rusting and rotting away on the outside.

There is no way around it. When you do not live life up to your purpose or exist without the requisite passion, you wake each day devoid of gratitude for the rebirth called today in word and deed.

You are rusting and rotting away. I was deteriorating and rotting away. I was not living up to my unlimited God-given potential.

But thank God, I received another chance to get it right. Thankfully, Naeem woke me up and reminded me that I could do more and that I still had time. And over the last many years, like the awards, honors, and recognitions show, I have done more with my precious gifted time.

Today, I'll do the same. I'll do more than I did with my life yesterday. I won't waste any time ever again.

On this day, I'll live my life with purpose and passion. I'll be the best version of myself possible. My gifts are out of the closet; there is no dust or rust in view. The talents the Creator gave me are all shiny and polished to present to others.

Thus, for whatever time remains, I'll present my gifts freely. My blessings will always be available to anyone who needs them and anyone who might find them helpful.

Reflect and Write:

Nate takes us back to where it all began, the genesis of this journal. In taking the time to remember how this journey began, he reflected, "But writing my son personalized letters was not intended to be an exhibition of excellent writing. The letters weren't supposed to be available for anyone but him. Yet writing him and then him electing to share the messages with others brought out a forgotten, buried part of me."

- What is a forgotten, buried part of you?

- What is something you once loved to do that you allowed life to push to the wayside?
- What gifts have you not offered to the world that only you possess?

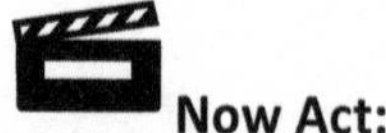
Now Act:

Thankfully, Naeem woke Nate up and reminded him that he could do more and that he still had time. Well, the same is true for you!

It's time to take those gifts out of the closet. Shake off the dust. Remove all the rust.

Today commit to pursuing something that you had buried deep. Today is the first day to do more with the time that you still have. Design a plan that includes one tangible thing you will do every day this week that moves you towards doing more with the time you still have available.

Journey Forward:

Week 12

Time to Love. No Regrets.

Good day, Journal,

We lost another great one today. Sadly, we lose great people every day. And like clockwork, when we lose folks, we have all so much to say about them. We set our social media pages ablaze.

When those we profess to love are no longer here, we can't seem to stop talking about how much they meant to us. But you know what, it's too late to talk about how much someone meant to you when that person is gone. You should have taken the time to shower them with your eternal love and devotion every opportunity you had while they were here. Nobody needed to hear and feel it more than those you proclaim to love who are now gone.

Yet, humans are just not that smart. Supposedly made in the Creator's image, yet the veracity of that statement seems more and more unlikely each day. We are a clueless bunch, every one of us—a people I often describe as the human family of Dumb and Dumber.

To put it simply, we don't know how to love. We have not even a little clue about what love means or how love should look insider or out.

Daily spouses and lovers part from each other, running out of the home like their hair is on fire, rushing to work where they spend most of their adult lives. They spend more time pouring their heart and soul into a career, most often working with people and for an organization that will never reciprocate their love than they do with their professed love.

And then one day, they get the unfortunate call that the person they promised to cherish for the rest of their life is gone. And of course, now they want everyone to know how much that person meant to them. Lamentably, the person who needed to be aware of their love, the person to convince, is gone. That person is dead and gone and can no longer hear loving words or feel the touch of a loved one.

The person for whom they spent their lifetime promising to get to them tomorrow, that person they always believed they could fit into their schedule later, is out of time. There are no more "laters," or afterward for them, when one is gone, together they are as a partnership or a family out of time.

Parents love their children the same way. Children love their parents no differently. The type of relationship is of no consequence. We undeniably don't know how to love people. We have no idea what it genuinely means to love one another.

It doesn't matter if it's spouses, moms and dads, children, friends, or extended family alike. We don't have a clue about what love legitimately means. None of us knows how to love.

Love is incomputable; it's invaluable; it's priceless. Yet, most of us think we can measure when we have sufficiently loved another or when we've paid an acceptable price for our loved one's time and energy—what a joke. Love is undoubtedly so much more than we give witness to in our pathetic words and feeble deeds.

Real love occurs when you give your time undividedly and your heart generously. You don't look at the clock. You aren't distracted by anything. You merely stay in the only moment that death teaches us that matters – the present, and you love passionately and intentionally.

Sadly, we all act as though love is easy. You merely say it, you make a couple of loving gestures, and you know and have agape like a Betty Crocker cake. I hate to tell you that's not what love is at all. A boxed cake does not make you a baker any more than loving gestures means you know how to love.

Love is everything; love is always and forever. Love is not optional; it's not one of those things you do when you feel like it. Love is not something that gets done when the time allows. Returning the deceased's love most certainly serves no one; it does no one any good when the person you can no longer say I love you to is dead and gone.

I sometimes feel like I'm preaching as though I am some evangelical pastor, but I'm not. I know, unfortunately, from experience what it means to proclaim you love someone and fail miserably. I loved a brother once, and I failed him so badly. He committed suicide, and regret has haunted me ever since.

I did not love him appropriately. I should have made more time for him. I should have known that he was not well mentally or emotionally. If I had loved him as the Creator commands me to love others, I believe he would be here today. Thus, each day, it is critical for me that I do not repeat that episode.

During the Pandemic, I talked to my mother via video call every single solitary day for months on end. There were days when I didn't want to do it, and then I remembered what it felt like to lose someone you love. If my mom were no longer, I would be begging God to give me more time with her. But the time we have today is all the time the Universe assures us of, so I called my mom, and I still call her every day to this day.

Every day during the Pandemic, I saw her face. Like the postal carrier, neither rain nor shine, nor sleet, nor snow stopped me. And I'm glad I did because it would be me having to live life with regret if something happened to her any of those months when all I had to do was take a moment to show and tell her I loved her.

And that's what love is today for most of us. That's how love gets reflected each time we lose someone. We call it 'love' when we lose someone, but in reality, the thing occurring, more often than not, with the loss of a loved one is regret. As I said, we don't know how to love, but we know how to experience remorse.

Today, I'll have no regrets. I will continue to give my attention undividedly and offer my time generously to those I love. Today, I'm going to love as if love really matters, as if I know something other folks don't seem to understand about time.

There are no promised tomorrow. If you do not love those, you proclaim to love with all your heart, soul, and mind immediately in the only moment you are guaranteed, the present, much sooner than later, you will only know regret in your heart, soul, and mind. And as I know all too well from my failure to love Terrell correctly, your heart, soul, and mind will only offer you a lifetime of regret.

Reflect and Write:

Nate shares how the loss of his dear friend, Terrell, taught him a valuable lesson about love and regrets. Re-read these two quotes from Nate. Be present. Fully present.

"Love is immeasurable; it's invaluable; it's priceless. Yet, most of us think we can measure when we have sufficiently loved another or when we've paid an acceptable price for our loved one's time and energy—what a joke. Love is undoubtedly so much more than we give witness to in our pathetic words and feeble deeds".

"Real love occurs when you give your time undividedly and your heart generously. You don't look at the clock. You aren't distracted by anything. You merely stay in the only moment that death teaches us that matters – the present, and you love passionately and intentionally."

Write your thoughts about love below.

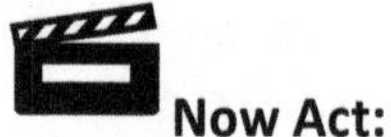

Now Act:

Now that you have written and reflected on love, to whom are you now prepared to commit to taking the time to love at this moment? How will you demonstrate this love? Will you make more time for the person? When you are next in their presence, which should happen soon, what steps will you take to give him/her/them your undivided attention? How much of your time will you offer? Who needs you to both tell and show them how much they mean to you? Pledge to have no regrets when this person is no longer with you.

Week 13

Naked Don't Lie

Good day, Journal,

It's been multiple decades now. But, it all began way back in December 1999 when I recognized if I didn't do something different about my health and fitness, I would not make it to see this day, much less any day in the distant future. Yes, that's when everything changed.

Two hundred and eleven plus pounds with an unimaginable body fat percentage. Unbelievable, as in I was unthinkably fat. Yeah, I was overweight, not big-boned.

Folks love to proclaim they are big-boned, but I have never seen a big-boned skeleton. All the bones I'd ever seen looked to be about the same composition. I didn't believe in big-boned skeletons; thus, there was no reason to continue BS'ing myself. I was fat, Pillsbury Dough Boy plump and soft.

But that was me before the new millennium. That was when my main man, my little man back then, unknowingly gifted me insight about who he desired to look up to. Naeem shared who he hoped to admire all the days of his life and the physical presence he expected his father to model forever.

Regrettably, the guy, my son sought did not yet exist. Sadly, only the overweight loving father was in the house, and that lard ass, 'Heavy Nate,' was me.

I was fat and delusional. But fortunately, I decided to start getting my health and fitness in order, given my child's guidance. Little did I know that the more attention I paid to my health, the more I concentrated on my fitness, the better everything in life became.

Changing how I saw myself and showed my appreciation for this leased Temple, the better everything in life became. I learned the divine truth behind the expression, "when you change, everything will change." When I changed my opinion of myself and showed it through my relentless commitment to be healthy and fit, everything about me changed.

People love to tell you that you look fine even when you know you look terrible underneath your expensive clothes. You know there are rows of fat and overlapping mounds of skin.

Still, it's crazy how you will pay more attention to the garment than you will do the flesh. It's absurd how we will starch and press our clothes to perfection but not count or sacrifice a calorie or push ourselves beyond physical mediocrity.

It's an absolute sham to believe that the clothes make the man or woman. What makes the man (woman) is the soul. The soul that is honest with itself makes the best of you.

The soul that is not afraid to tell you that you are not living as the Creator designed you who gets you to become the best version of yourself possible. The soul that yells to you, "You look terrible, and you need to get your house in both internal and external order," is doling out the cold-hearted truth making a great human.

Please beware and be on the lookout for those folks who often proclaim that you look fine when you know better. Putting lovely drapes on the window of a junky house does not mean the home is no longer junky. Clothing is no different.

Clothes are the drapes that hide what you know exists on the inside and underneath. In my case, clothes hid that I treated the Temple leased to me by the Creator, not like the Holy Sanctuary it deserved. Instead, I treated the Temple like a low rent high-rise apartment.

The Temple assigned to me came initially in the condition of a newly constructed pristine Taj Mahal. But, sadly, I treated it; I made it over the years look like Cabrini-Green, a community of dilapidated condemned row houses.

Now back to those folks who tell you look fine when you know you don't. They aren't honestly telling you that you look fine. Please don't be so gullible. No way are they complimenting you.

Journey Forward:

What's meant in truth is that they don't want to do more with their lives, and they don't want to feel pressured to do so by your improvement. So, if you treat your Temple like Motel 6 or Super 8, they get to do the same. They can remain as you used to exist, 'fat and happy.'

They claim to want better, but they aren't willing to do better. Most people dwell in the 'Fool's Paradise,' and if possible, they want you to keep living in that fantasy world right alongside them as well.

Sometimes, when you decide to be better, you become the mirror that others view their reflection. Often you turn into that great humanity beacon, saying it's time for them to change and do more and be better. At times, you are the flashing brightly beaming neon sign that says, "Naked, don't lie, stop being a liar!"

Don't lie to yourself today. Don't lie to yourself ever again. Instead, each morning, do whatever is required to be the best version of yourself possible. Get on the scale, do it naked and watch as the truth appears right before your eyes live, in living color, and with digital precision.

One-hundred, seventy-eight pounds, 10 percent body fat. Yes, indeed. That's what the scale reads, and I'll add the rest. I'm 178 pounds of twisted steel with young Denzel chocolate sex appeal. Best of all, if it weren't against the law, I could stay naked all day, every day. But I digress!

Nevertheless, for sure, I don't need expensive drapes to look good these days, nor is there anything about me I want to hide or that I'm afraid of others seeing. I'm 178 pounds of twisted steel with young Denzel chocolate sex appeal. I'm abundantly wealthy and in mental possession of timeless wisdom.

My life is as I imagined precisely. Because long ago, I accepted the truth that naked, be it mental, physical, or spiritual, don't lie; only people do. People are lying savants; I was a lying guru once upon a time as well. But not anymore.

Thanks to my man in training, I understood that it was past time to stop lying to myself. Thanks to my main man, I'm living the life I always imagined because I know better than ever to fear or be embarrassed by being naked – mind, body, or soul. Today, I'm living my best life because I'm stark raving naked.

Reflect and Write:

"When I changed my opinion of myself and showed it through my relentless commitment to be healthy and fit, everything about me changed."

"In my case, clothes hid that I treated the Temple leased to me by the Creator, not like the Holy Sanctuary it deserved. Instead, I treated the Temple like a low rent high rise apartment."

Do your actions reflect your opinion of yourself? What do you need to do to ensure that your actions align for your best life as Nate's actions now align with his child's guidance and thoughts?

Are you treating your body like the limited edition that it is? If not, why? Now that you have identified your excuse, it's time to create an action plan.

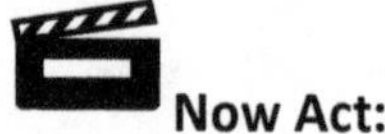

Now Act:

Say this to yourself three times: "I accept the truth that naked, be it mental, physical, or spiritual, don't lie; only people do."

What lies have you been telling yourself about your health and wellness? Whatever they are, the lies stop today.

Write down your 21-day commitment to be healthy and fit. Start tomorrow. Keep a journal. Find an accountability partner (one who will not lie). We will check back with you in 3 weeks (21 days).

Journey Forward:

Week 14

Tired

Good day, Journal,

Am I tired! Boy, am I ever! My middle name could be 'tired,' given the degree to which exhaustion plays a role in my life. But no matter what I call this feeling drained, exhausted, weary, or tired, it doesn't matter.

It just doesn't matter if I'm tired. Nobody cares about you being tired. People only care about results. Those who are waiting on you to help, serve and make sure they know that their life matters are exhausted too. The "least of these" are far more depleted than you.

So, each day, you need to suck it up, period. There is no time for whining or feeling sorry for yourself. You got to get going because being tired doesn't truly matter; it must not matter anymore.

When you were a child, you would tell your dad that you were tired, and his words were usually of the variety, "Boy if you don't get up and do something, I'll give you something for which to be tired." The thing he promised to give was a spanking. I got up immediately because he was right. A spanking made me tired. Sick and tired. Genuinely exhausted, I was with him being my father and treating me this way.

Despite the harshness of his words and the rudeness of his behavior, I've learned to embrace the spirit of his remarks. When you aren't up and doing good, leaving you tired at the end of the day, this life has consequences for choosing rest over labor. This life can give you experiences that will leave you weary.

Perhaps that's why I'm always working. Why I'm forever writing something, continuously pondering the next big thing—continually trying to get my mind to rest so that I can be less tired. But no such luck for me. I'm stuck being in a perpetual state of exhaustion.

Like Dr. King's "I've Been to the Mountaintop" speech, when it comes to being tired, I'll state over and again emphatically, "it doesn't matter to me anymore; I've been to the resting place before." On the other side is rest, and to be honest, the other place, resting, scares me more than where I am now.

When I think about rest, I mostly imagine the final resting place, the other side of life where I know I'll be kicking and screaming in opposition to the Creator's answer, begging and pleading with the Universe for more time. I suspect I'll be asking the Universe like a spoiled brat for just a bit more time because I hadn't done everything I hoped to do. And the Universe will nonchalantly respond in the voice of Tommie L. Turner, "you have no more time, you should have spent more time doing and less time resting."

And with that outlook, it looks like I'm going to be tired yet again today. I do not want to live a life of regrets. It is not my plan to reach the final resting place and find a reason to calculate when I wasted all my moments when I could have been doing what is required to live my best life that I spent resting.

Yeah, we all need to rest now and again. A good night's sleep does the mind, body, and soul well. But given the choice of a good night's sleep or a great life, a life of meaning, an existence of purpose, an opportunity to leave the planet better than it was when I arrived, I will most certainly always choose being tired.

Yes, indeed, I'm tired. I'm so very exhausted, and I couldn't be happier. Being dog-tired is what made me who I am today. Being worn out is how I stay in excellent health, maintain abundant wealth, and possess timeless wisdom.

I'm tired, yes! But I'm never tired of living my life precisely as I do, just as I always imagined.

Reflect and Write:

Nate is as busy as this journal reflects. His mind is always going. He is always moving. And being tired is something to which we all can relate. However, the question we must answer is, "What is the fruit that comes as a result of our tiredness?"

Journey Forward:

Nate tells us, "I do not want to live a life of regrets. It is not my plan to reach the final resting place and find a reason to calculate all the time I wasted all the moments when I could have been doing what is required to live my best life that I spent resting."

When you rest from your work, is it work that has placed you on the path toward the life you always wanted to live?

Does your tiredness come from being busy but not being productive?

What type of tired are you? Mentally? Physically? Emotionally? Is it leading you to a place of fulfillment or just passing time?

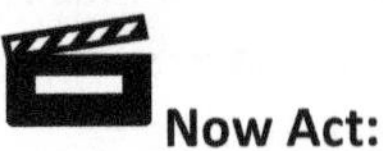

Now Act:

Are you tired? Daily make a list of the things you do that lead you to be tired. Are there things on the list to be eliminated because they are not leading you towards the life you want to live?

This week pick one item from the list to eliminate once and for all. At the end of the week, revisit this journal entry and reflect on how you feel. Once you come back to this journal entry, identify a second item to eliminate. Come back as often as you need to until you have replaced the empty things that are causing you to be fatigued with those that propel you towards your best life.

Week 15

Mad as Hell

Good day, Journal,

Sometimes when I look back to COVID-19, I get angry all over again. And to be clear, being angry is something for which this Black man is well known. Yet, I'm not mad for some unimportant or trivial reason.

I'm mad for things like the stupidity of Americans that believed wearing a mask and social distancing was an infringement on their civil liberties. Living in such a divisive nation where citizens prefer to choose sides for every matter when segregating is entirely unnecessary pisses me off.

I'm sick and tired of being guided by a nation of dumb and dumber political, governmental, and corporate leaders. The Dumb and Dumber leaders, as I refer to them, that cause the rest of us to live a real-life 'Ground Hog – This Is the Worst Day Ever' existence.

I'm angry at much stuff. I'm perturbed by several people. Still, mostly, I'm mad because people wouldn't listen to me earlier.

Let me get this right out in the open; my frustration is not an issue of ego. Hell, we all have egos, but I keep mine in check most of the time, unlike the masses. I know that kind of sounds like I have an ego.

When it comes to helping, serving, and making sure others know that their life matters, all that matters to me is helping, serving, and making sure others know that they matter. I don't give a damn about being right or being rewarded.

Whether I get any credit for helping, serving, and making sure others know their life matters is, unequivocally, of no importance to me. Trust me when I tell you, any credit I get is irrelevant; credit to me will always be superfluous.

I only want to help, serve, and make sure others know that their life matters. I want to give back some of the blessings and goodness long associated with my life. Let me restate; I must give back. The Universe demands that I pay it (the Celestial grace and Cosmic mercy extended undeservingly to me) forward.

My life is fantastic. Look around and see for yourself. I'm in excellent health, maintain abundant wealth, and possess timeless wisdom. Did I mention that I'm still 178 pounds of twisted steel with young Denzel chocolate sex appeal at my age? Please don't make me show off my six-pack. Yes, abs, I don't drink beer.

But I digress. My life should not be amazing alone. I don't ever want to be the aberration, the statistical anomaly. I've been the statistical anomaly before, and it's an overrated experience.

Instead, I want all humans to enjoy life experiences equal to or superior to mine. My preference, my great desire, is that all humans will share in the opportunity to enjoy life, liberty, and the pursuit of happiness equally without infringement. This declared independence is not only what I will hope for but what I promise to work towards for others all the days of my life.

Thus, I'm so pissed off because we could have saved hundreds of thousands of lives. We could have ensured that students, especially those already subjects of substandard education, did not fall further behind in the Fourth Industrial Revolution's world measurement of college and career readiness. We could have reduced, if not eliminated, the housing inequities and all the associated standards of living inequalities that haunt the unhoused and the socio-demographically marginalized in America.

I tried to share my ideas with everyone who would hear me out: strategies about the changing landscape of business, schools, and homes. I offered a plan that would have reduced the spread of COVID all over this nation, particularly throughout historically marginalized and underserved neighborhoods.

I started talking about the nano-community long before the pandemic. A new society comprised of small self-contained, economically self-sufficient, energy-independent, green-spaced, and diverse neighborhoods. Specialized communities where social status was irrelevant, where the best of humanity extended to the treatment of all humans.

I shared an idea for learning in the 21st century. A concept that began with prepared parents who could authentically be as we proclaim parents to be children's first teachers. A neighborhood with nano-community schools at the heart of the locale built to net-zero standards and reduced funding dependence on zip codes and property tax.

Finally, there would be an academic institution where mastery of subject matter rather than rote learning was the essential scholastic ingredient to intellectual growth. An educational system that prepared parents in a Lamaze, Google maps, meet the Khan Academy approach. An innovative, disruptive methodology based on long-term thinking to raise a nation of intellectually ambitious, globally, and culturally competent, humanitarian-driven citizens.

Finally, a real education not one steeped in 19th-century assembly line worker tradition and antiquated model-T origin. No, a modern-day, best, and next-level practice approach preparing the future to be better and brighter because our children were genuinely improved and more radiant by all international measurements.

Alas, they didn't listen. The 'powers that be' believed they knew better; they thought themselves smarter than me. But you were wrong; you didn't know more than me. For the record, you still aren't more intelligent than me.

The world suffered unnecessarily. The residents of the planet still suffer today. And for which, I'm still mad as hell!

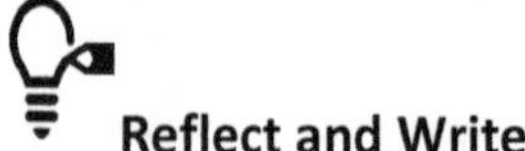

Reflect and Write:

What makes you mad as hell? Seriously, write it down.

Now that you have gotten that out in the open and off your chest, what solutions do you have? Seriously, you know you have ideas, so write them down.

I know that you, like Nate, want all humans (even if it's just the humans in your home) to enjoy life experiences equal to or superior to yours. So, what are you going to do about it? Who can you tell? Who can you engage to help you bring about the change you know is necessary?

Journey Forward:

Now Act:

Look back at your list of things that make you mad as hell. Select one of the things and create action steps to eradicate it. Remember, the only action that is too small is inaction. Please, commit to doing something for the next seven days that address that thing that makes you mad.

Week 16

Re-centered

Good day, Journal,

Finally! I've arrived. It seems like it took forever to get here. No, I'm not talking about the arduous road to becoming an award-winning author and renowned public intellectual. I'm merely talking about the flight from L.A.X. to Fiji.

I love to travel, but I'm not a big fan of these long flights. A large plane weighs so much staying up in the air for so long seems simply wrong. But the aircraft, like my life, does the unbelievable. With the grace and mercy of the Creator, the plane and my life make what appears impossible on the surface authentically and incontrovertibly palpable.

The lengthy travel required to get away from my daily life is, I suppose, the price one must pay to go somewhere where they've never been but longed to go. Again, the flight was much like my life – an extended journey featuring lots of turbulence to finally arrive where I always wanted to be.

Yes, I'm on top of the literary world right now. With the overwhelming success of "The Amazing World of STEM" series, I'm also on top of many other worldwide categories such as film, social commentary, and amusement parks. And strangely, even when I gratefully reflect on all the imagination and effort it took to finally succeed, I find myself wanting to get away from it all. I want to get away for at least a short while.

Now this moment is so simple and, yes, incredible all at the same time. The Pacific Ocean is playing the soundtrack to the moment. As I lay in the sand, waves go to and from the deep ocean to the nearby shore. The sound is unbelievable. Relaxing and reassuring are the rhythmic pulsation of the water.

Hearing the waves reminds me that I am alive. Like a heartbeat, the tides seem to throb, as is the case when a medical professional takes your pulse.

Journey Forward:

The air is fresh. Perhaps as fresh as any place that I've ever visited. The fresh air is a reminder of the freshness of each new day, the fresh daily outlook that one must have if they plan to get through the tossing and turning of life's salty wave-like dimensions.

It's the same Pacific Ocean as the one I walk out to each day from my home, but it's somewhat different from my Pacific Ocean at the same time. No one knows me here. No one even cares to know me or my name. Here I am as I believe myself to be always no one, nobody.

Here there are no putting on airs or false flattery. When the indigenous people here speak to you, they do so from the best of humanity, not because they desire anything from you. When the native folks communicate with you here, they merely exhibit a genuine empathy for a fellow human. The human spirit here is honest and beautiful.

I love my home and my country, and at the same time, I grow weary of the so-called 'Land of the Free.' With significant accomplishments and realized dreamt recognitions comes a decreased level of freedom.

My present, the time gifted to me by the Creator, more and more are less my own. Even my desire to help, serve and make sure others know that their life matters is often interrupted. Impacted routinely is my life by things that are nowadays beyond my control.

I now have media requests that I didn't have before. I now have publicity demands that were not a part of my life previously. Now that I'm no longer broke and 'money ain't a thang,' I have more people than one could imagine trying their best to grab my bag. Folks come out of the woodwork now routinely attempting to find out just how fat and deep my pockets are in reality.

But I'm rambling unnecessarily. My mind is wandering discourteously! I've started to lose focus of all that the Universe makes available for me, what's important about life, and living in this moment.

I'm not here to focus on where I was. I'm here to get my mind right to regroup. My time here is about getting re-centered to resume living my best life. To realign my trinity to continue envisioning a seemingly impossible life and make that life inevitable. Now is my time to prepare for the tremendous and never-ending fight to leave the planet better when I depart than it was upon my arrival.

Ah, the waves. The water rushing towards the shore is so glorious. Lying on my back in the sand with the water rushing up to my feet is all the reminder I need that my life is fantastic. Thank you, Source, for this remarkable life. Namaste!

Reflect and Write:

The quest for your best life can be a grind. We all must take time to recenter and regroup. You may not be able to hop on a flight to Fiji (just yet), but you can and should take time to recenter.

Nevertheless, you can take a moment to think about what actions best help you calibrate after long stretches of focus and effort towards your goals. Write down a list of where you go and what you do whenever you find yourself losing focus.

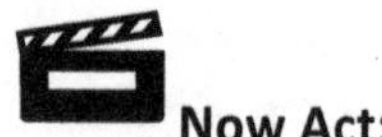

Now Act:

Decide right now to do something this week to refuel and recharge. Be specific. Set an appointment with yourself. Put the scheduled time with yourself in your calendar. Most importantly, keep and make the meeting.

Even if it's just 60 minutes, keep your promise to yourself. Follow through precisely as you have been encouraged to do right now. The time is now, and this is the moment for you to get into the never-ending fight to leave the planet better when you depart than it was upon your arrival.

Week 17

Hunger

Good day, Journal,

There is no liberation to be found lying in bed. The only thing you are likely to find in bed is yesterday's burdens. Included in your mattress are all the mental and emotional things draining you of the Universe's bounteous promise called today.

You will never live, not one day of life, as you always imagined if you continue to sleep your life away. So, get up now. Mentally, physically, and spiritually, get your ass up now and get going immediately. Get up because your best life waits for no one, not even you!

Such I know is true. I know this is valid because my friend and mentor, Les Brown, told me so. "You gotta be hungry!" Yes, you must be hungry! Not hungry as in "yeah, I could eat." Not hungry as in "pinch me off a corner, I'll have a taste." Not hungry as in "well, just let me see if I like how it tastes first."

Nope, to get the life you always wanted to live your best life experiences day in and day out, you must be more than a little ambitious. You must have a voracious insatiable appetite for greatness. You gotta be hungry! (said with belly-aching emphasis)

And when you are hungry, when your tummy is growling, and the pain of not having eaten is unremittingly upon you, the one thing you cannot do for sure is sleep. You cannot sleep when you are hungry. You cannot think straight when you are hungry.

Nothing, and I do mean nothing, means anything when you are hungry. Nothing works as it's supposed to when you are hungry. Your mind goes blank, your body has no energy for movement, and your soul seems empty.

You will know the Les Brown version of hunger when the only thing that matters, the singular thing that matters above all things in those depleted moments, is getting something to eat. Consuming whatever is missing from your life ravenously and insatiably.

That's how you got here. That's how you write and publish award-winning and best-selling books so prolifically. That's how you write and give speeches with the Celestial speed of light and the Cosmic gift of gab with Divine ease.

It's how your words and deeds are known and celebrated by others ubiquitously throughout the world. It's how you purchased this beach home with cash. It's how you remain in excellent health, enjoy abundant wealth, and possess timeless wisdom.

Staying hungry is an undeserved gift from the Source so that you will never disobey your call to help, serve, and make sure others know that their life matters daily. Your life's outward blessings originate from the inward instructions to stay hungry to find a continuous way to starve internally, even when you appear externally satisfied.

You get to do more because you remain hungrier than most. You will continue to do more than most, not because you are bigger, better, or brighter. Your brilliance is simply obedience wrapped inside the realization that you must remain hungry. "You gotta be hungry!" It would be best if you felt the pain of insatiable starvation all the time.

But how does one remain insatiably hungry? How do you feel the pains of unappeasable starvation when all sorts of life's filling and satisfying creature comforts abound? You merely ask and answer for yourself any one of these questions:

- 'Have I done all that I could ever do with my life?'
- 'Am I living each gloriously gifted moment to my full potential?
- 'Is there anything or anyone, my talents, or my gifts could benefit that I have yet assisted?'

Should any of the answers connote an incompleteness, if there is the slightest twinge of self-satisfaction it means, you haven't accomplished anything at all! Until you can say, you've done all I can do with your life, that you're living all moments to your fullest God-given potential, and that there is nothing or no one who needs to be helped, served, or made to know that their life matters you know you have work to do.

Until there is no hunger, mental, physical, or spiritual, anywhere, I know there is no time for me to rest. If there is hunger anywhere in the world, I know I gotta be hungry.

Reflect and Write:

"You must have a voracious insatiable appetite for greatness." Does this statement describe you? Let's look at the questions Nate posed in today's journal. Take a moment and honestly reflect on each question. How you answer each of these will determine what you do next.

- 'Have I done all that I could ever do with my life?'
- 'Am I living each gloriously gifted moment to my full potential?'
- 'Is there anything or anyone, my talents, or my gifts could benefit that I have yet assisted?'

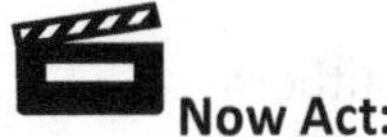

Now Act:

Choose at least one of the questions above where your answer was negative where you acknowledge you could do more. Give some thought to what more you can do.

Then start a list of what would have to happen for you to answer the question in the affirmative, as in you've done everything humanly possible. Identify one of those items from your list and start doing more today!

Week 18

Unstuck

Good day, Journal,

Another one! Almost as if DJ Khaled were here in the flesh in my beach house broadcasting the weather, I imagine him saying "another one" over and over again. Another one, as in today, is another beautiful Southern California January day. Another day in the low to mid-70s. I believe that's five days in a row.

And to think, I almost didn't make it out here. For a long time, I believed my sentence was to live out my remaining days in Indiana. As if I existed in some real-life purgatory, I thought myself a man destined to remain in Indiana.

Yep, you heard that correctly – Indy-freaking-ana. I know! I know! I agree absolutely!

The words Indiana and Nate don't go together at all. Nate's from Indiana doesn't roll off the tongue like Nate's from Cal-I-Forn-I-A! Nate's from (say it fast with rhythm) California!

Seriously, my internal design, my spiritual innards, is to live in Southern California. I think Southern California was waiting for my arrival all the time. From the tip of my head to the soul of my feet, Southern California and I share a kindred connection.

Sure, great people lived in California before I arrived. Undoubtedly, there will be many great folks here after I'm gone. Still, the State needed me as much, if not more, than I needed it.

Or at least that's what I like to tell myself every morning. It's how I reconcile the ridiculous cost of living on the Pacific Ocean coast. Yeah, Southern California needed me to be here. Yep! That's my story, and I'm sticking to it.

Ultimately, I finally got out of Indiana thanks to recognizing that I could no longer allow the dream of a perfect outcome to be an obsession that kept me from following good ideas. My mind and soul left Indiana long ago. At last, my body was able to finally arrive to join my mind and soul in Southern California.

That's how I made the physical trek to California to live out the next stage of the journey called life. Not long ago, I was stuck. I'm telling you, I was stuck thinking that life had to be perfect before I could do something good.

But I am stuck no more. Now I understand that what we believe is a "perfect life" is genuinely just a life of more good moments than bad moments.

There is no perfect life, after all. Believing we can ever be infallible is the lie that keeps us from doing good. As the Italian philosopher, Voltaire said, "perfect is the enemy of good."

Of course, humans should strive for perfection. Still, we must never let the fear of not achieving perfection keep us from giving our all – deter us from trying our best every time.

Foolishly, too many of us want things to be perfect before we try to do anything at all. We let the desire for perfection keep us from living a good life, even missing out on our best life experiences.

In my early years, I failed to change my life because I wanted to be perfect. Because of all those useless attempts to be perfect, I missed many good opportunities, far too many good moments to count.

Long ago, I waited for the perfect time to write a book to discover that the best time to write is when the book first appears in your mind, not when you have a major publisher in the wings. Long ago, I waited for the perfect time to document my good idea about reimagining communities. I foolishly believed that an expert in community development needed to validate my opinion but was I ever wrong.

Today, I realize that right now is the time to do what you believe needs doing. Now is absolutely the right time to pursue the life you always imagined. You don't need the time to be perfect; you only need to act with good intentions and great effort right now.

Before I was 178 pounds of twisted steel with young Denzel chocolate sex appeal, I was "198 pounds of crumpled aluminum with Old Denzel 'Fences' mocha sex repellant." That means my health and fitness were an insult to the Creator. I was certainly not treating the gift of flesh and bone as the wondrous elements making up this gloriously gifted Temple for which I possess.

Yet, instead of waiting for the perfect time to get my ass in shape, I started where I was so that I could finally be who I wanted to be. Today, I'm 178 pounds..., and most days, I look so good; I want to jump back and kiss myself. Muah!

No, I don't consider myself perfect, but I give my best effort daily. I devote an excellent attempt each moment the Universe gifts me to be as close to perfect as possible. That's what perfection is all about anyway. Giving all that we have 'in all present moments' to be as close to perfect as possible is perfection.

And while perfect may be humanly unattainable, it should not and must not keep us, humans, from giving our all. I may not be perfect, but that won't ever stop me from giving all that I have to help, serve, and make sure all people know that their life matters.

Nope, I probably won't ever be perfect, I may not even know what an ideal day looks like, but that won't stop me from trying to be perfect. And now, as if I'm DJ Khaled repeating the phrase for which he is best known over and over and over again, "another one."

Another (one) day to give my all to do my best to live the life I always imagined. Another (one) chance not to let perfection be the enemy of the good. Another (one) opportunity to experience a nice moment, a terrific day, my best life.

Reflect and Write:

The fear of not being perfect was once a hindrance for Nate, but then he got unstuck. What has been keeping you from giving your all? What deters you from trying your best every time?

Get a piece of paper. Make a list of what and where you are stuck. Be honest. Remember being honest with yourself is part of the reason why you journal.

Journey Forward:

Your journal is the place for you to get out of your way and move forward towards your best life.

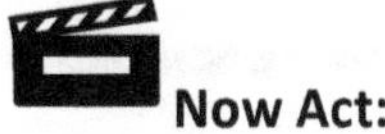

Now Act:

Take the list of things keeping you stuck and rip it up. They are just artificial, false barriers you created and don't deserve any more energy anyway.

The way to get unstuck is to start where you are right now simply. What will you get up and begin doing immediately to move you towards your best life?

It doesn't have to be some grand, sweeping gesture. If you are on a quest like Nate to get to your version of 178 pounds twisted steel with young Denzel sex appeal, you can get unstuck by merely going for a walk RIGHT now. Whatever it is you've identified as something to help you get unstuck, don't delay. Do that thing or things now.

Week 19

Persevere

Good day, Journal,

Top of the day to you, Great Spirit. I hear you loud and clear. Today take no interest in being courageous. Instead, focus solely on the fear and disappointment associated with not having done all you can do to be the best version of yourself.

I entirely concur a pinch of perseverance beats a cup of courage regularly. As if you are holding the winning hand in poker, perseverance is the royal flush that beats every hand. I know this to be unequivocally true. Perseverance tops courage every time, all the time.

Generally, folks get it all wrong believing greatness requires courage or that, as an example, the dialogue that changes the world is "courageous conversations." Not true at all. What brings excellence forth and makes words life and world-changing are the deeds those persevering actions.

I tell those who will listen that my genius, if there is any in my possession, is that I operate from a place of fear. I live on the bank of disappointment. Daily, when I arise, I rise to do great things, not out of courage. I rise to the occasion because of the elixir called perseverance, a composition of fear and disappointment.

I am fearful of not living up to my potential. I don't want to disappoint those counting on me to help, serve, and ensure no one doubts that all life matters. Thus, I persevere. I keep moving forward, no matter what.

Courage is a fascinating attribute. We all have the quality, but so few want to do the work it takes to initiate one of humanity's chief features.

Courage is like that old-school gas-powered lawnmower that you must pull the cord hard precisely unerring to get the lawnmower to start. Perseverance: fear and disappointment are altogether different.

Journey Forward:

Everyone has an intimate relationship with fear and disappointment. Fear and disappointment are effortless attributes to ignite. They are the mulching lawnmower where all you must do is push and walk. To activate the power of fear and disappointment takes almost no energy or thought at all.

While born with little doubt, babies get delivered to the earth with two innate fears: the fear of falling and loud sounds. We are not born courageous. Courage is a developed quality, a characteristic that comes with a certain amount of pain and loathing, anguish, and aversion that the multitude would preferably escape.

Courage is one of the most contrived human behaviors. To be courageous requires one to do something uniquely unnatural to draw on the Supernatural. And yet, we want the benefits of courage without being audacious. Such aspirations and expectations are both illogical and unreasonable.

I'm no different, which is why fear and disappointment normally power my life. I don't want to meet the Creator and find myself explaining why I didn't work harder to live life as I imagined. I don't wish for the Source to interrogate me on that final day about why I didn't live my life to its fullest. I don't want to be grilled until I am ready to testify that I road my day-to-day experiences until the wheels of life fell off.

On a human note, I don't want to see the look of disappointment in the eyes of those who love and adore me should I not give my all to be the best I can be. Again, there is nothing courageous about this process. Built on fear and disappointment is my strategy for living my best life. I move forward simply because I persevere.

Today, I will allow fear and disappointment to fuel me to aid me to be better than I was yesterday. Fear and disappointment, the twins of greatness shall make it appear that I am courageous even though, in truth, I am not.

I will persevere today as I've done all the days before today. Everyone who lived yesterday and who has breath in their lungs now knows perseverance—all living beings preserved through yesterday to today. A small sampling of living beings exhibited courage, but most of us merely persevered.

Most of us who accomplished anything worth noting yesterday did so by taking advantage of fear and disappointment. Today will be much the same.

I will remain fearful of disappointing those who love and adore me. I will keep moving forward. I will persevere through the virtuous and evil moments. I will endure because I have no interest in explaining to the Universe why I didn't do what the Source called me to do. I do not intend to ask for forgiveness for not leaving the planet better upon my departure than upon my arrival.

I will persevere. I will stay fearful. What will drive me is not wanting to disappoint.

Reflect and Write:

What fuels you? What is the "why" of your existence, your reason for being? What will cause you to keep going even when the going gets tough?

Take time today to write yourself a letter. Tell your next year self what your life looks like in 365 days because you kept going, because you persevered.

Now Act:

Place the letter you wrote in an envelope. Address the envelope, seal it, and place a stamp on it. Give the envelope to a reliable friend or loved one. Ask him/her/them to mail it to you in precisely 365 days. Set an alert in your phone to remember to remind them not to forget to send the letter.

Now get to work making what you wrote in that letter your reality.

Week 20

A Spark

Good day, Journal,

Just one drop. That's all you need is one drop of possibility, only one piece of hope. That's all you need to make this life your best life.

Unfortunately, some people incorrectly believe that you need the glass to be half full to see the potential in the day. But not you. You don't need any of that to see the present promise staring you smack dab in the face.

You know, don't you! You know something others do not know. With a Cheshire cat grin on your face, you understand that all it takes is for a speck of hope to exist to make today the first day the best day in the life you always imagined.

Long ago, don't you remember you shared with Naeem the idea about the glass that appeared virtually empty? Only it wasn't void. Inside, the crystal was a speck of bread. The glass, unwashed and left to sit, eventually grew to a glass with mold everywhere. Mold grew nonstop inside and outside the glass. There was little to no limit to the prodigious growth of the mold.

And this is what hope looks like for you. Such is the way you must always embrace the interminable possibility of your life.

Daily, it would be best to remember that even when things appear darkest when all hope seems lost, the fact that you awoke this morning and that you are alive right now means you are like that speck of bread in the glass. Of course, I don't mean to imply that you are stinky and toxic, like overgrown mold.

I mean that inside you is the potential to grow to untold levels mainly because you believe that it doesn't take a glass to be half full to succeed. Instead, you know that you merely need there to be a speck, even the most minuscule glimpse of a possibility.

The wisest and most accomplished would say that is what makes this life extraordinary. We don't need a glass to be half full to succeed. Suppose we follow a process that sets things in motion, and we are willing to remain patient. In that case, the unbelievable can be made believable.

But it would help if you stayed patient. Not patient as a definition of lazy but patient as in remaining steady, following the script day after day, staying on course without deviating from the process, and continuously abiding by a celebrated procedure with an illustrious history of success. Believing not because you hope it will work. Imagining because you know in your heart and mind that all things are possible for any who believes with words and bangs and clangs with deeds at their craft relentlessly.

Today, I no longer need a half-full glass to know that the life I always imagined living is a possibility and that my best life is inevitable. I understand that the speck is like a spark, and both are synonymous with me.

A spark in a dry forest is all that is required to set the forest ablaze. One tiny spark can do more damage than most could imagine; that is everyone other than the spark.

The spark knows its potential, and it knows that all it must do is wait patiently to stay ready and not need to get prepared for when the time is right. And when that day comes and the forest is at its driest, and the wind starts to blow precisely accurate, that spark begins saying the mantra to itself "wait for it, wait for it."

The spark's chant is its reminder, its call to action to wait for the sun to shine at the appropriate temperature and angle. And poof shazam, when the moment is ideal, the spark is lit, and the dry forest begins to burn and burn uncontrollably.

I don't want any forest to burn up or anyone to be sickened by mold. Still, I want you to stay mindful and remain alert to the truth that it only takes something small to make life big.

Today, I will do the small things with precision, and I will do them exceedingly well. Today, I will not rush the process because doing so would lessen my internal growth, outer reach, and impact on the world.

Journey Forward:

I am the spark. I am the mold like penicillin that will leave the planet better when I depart than when I arrived.

Staying prepared for my opportunity, I will do. Believing that the glass is always some full portion will make it possible for me to live up to my unlimited God-given potential. Following the behavior of the mold and the spark will allow me to best help, serve, and make sure countless others know that their life matters.

Reflect and Write:

What small things have you done over the last 20 weeks that have proved to be the sparks to move you towards your best life?

Spend some extended time today reading back over your journal entries. Celebrate even the small things that you have done exceedingly well.

Embrace the process. Look at how you have changed. Note how your life is better than it was when you first opened this journal.

Consider what small things you can begin doing today that will keep you moving forward. Write it here. Remember, it just takes a spark.

Now Act:

Write the one thing that could be your spark and place it in a prominent place in your home, somewhere you will see it every day. Commit to doing this one thing well for the next 22 weeks. You won't regret it.

Week 21

Control

Good day, Journal,

Ladies and gentlemen, what a pleasure it is to be here with you today. Thank you so very much for accepting the invitation to join us.

I'm so grateful that you chose to spend some of your time here today with me. You could have been doing anything else or traveled to any other location in the world today. Still, you chose to fill up this auditorium to hear me speak.

The 2020 election, wow! That's where I'll start and remain most of this lecture. Let me repeat it. Wow!

Does anyone remember 2020? That's a joke, folks. Who can ever forget 2020? I don't think we could erase 2020 from our memories if we tried. I don't think anyone could force themselves to forget 2020, even if we could voluntarily get Alzheimer's or Dementia.

From COVID-19 to social unrest, economic turmoil, and the options for political candidates ranging from morbid to catastrophic, 2020 was quite simply a pain in the ass. I'm not usually one for looking ahead or living beyond the present, but I must tell you, 2020 tried my patience. Like you, I was ready to escape the moment and send 2020 packing.

I remember on November 3rd, going to bed relatively early, at least early for me. It was around 10:30 pm. I refused to watch any news or anything political. Hell, I figured what was the point anyway. I had my suspicions about which of the two candidates would win. Besides, the news coverage was like a sport, comparable to following a tennis match and bad for sleeping.

Each consecutive minute the commentator was doing their best to volley our emotions and mental state like two tennis pros playing against one another. One minute the ball was in one candidate's court; then it was in the other candidate's court, then one person was up a game, then things were even. It was too much intentional emotional distress for any one person, so I went to bed.

I knew when I woke; I would rise to morbidity or catastrophe. Either way, when I got out of bed, I was sure this Nation would still be a complete mess. Yes, I would wake up still a citizen in The U.S.A., The Unmitigated States of Acrimony.

I woke before 5 am. I finally got out of bed around 5:20 am with a feeling of foreboding in the pit of my stomach. And as was the case before I went to bed, I refused to look at the news. I did not turn on anything electronic. I avoided being the bouncy tennis ball bounced to and fro in the match of no-good options.

What I did that morning was the part of this horrendous story that I want you to hold on to as the only truth for which you can and should ever depend. I got out of bed grateful, appreciative, and encouraged because it is what the Universe demands of me daily.

I did not speak a word. I went to the restroom, brushed my teeth with my left hand. I'm right-handed, but using my left hand activates my brain. I walked into the kitchen, mixed 6 ounces of water with 6 ounces of cranberry concentrate. I swallowed a caffeine pill with a tablespoon of psyllium husk; my colon, like the day, deserved a fresh start.

Then I went downstairs, opened my laptop to write in my Journal. In the spirit of the voting season, I elected to remain consistent with my process. Living my best life requires appreciating my only life, "living in the moment" daily.

As I have done now for years, I wrote about my best life as I imagined living it regardless of the news; I would learn in 30 minutes or so. What the Nation decided or, more accurately, which of the two horrendous options it settled on was of little consequence. The Universe's mission for me would be unchanged. My charge to help, serve and make sure others know their lives mattered would remain no matter who America settled on as President.

There in the dark of the early morning, I remembered that we could only control what we can control. Each morning, when the good Lord wakes me in my right mind, which is undoubtedly questionable fiction for some, I have but one voluntary choice to make. I can choose to be present to live my best life today or elect to be somewhere else, most notably in a previous day, a past day for which I have no power to change.

The election, especially in 2020, featuring a decaying democracy, affirmed just how powerless we are to do anything more than be the best version of ourselves possible. The election, all elections but particularly the 2020 election, set me on the course and seemingly did the same for you to learn to pivot and iterate to be better Americans who work together to genuinely create a "more perfect union."

Together we have learned to change what we can change. While we are not yet capable of changing the entire Nation in some small ways, we have done just that. It's in part why we are gathered here today in mass. Today, we celebrate that we are nothing like the typical American.

Look at how many nano-communities now exist—thriving tiny nation-states within a crumbling oxymoronic misnamed "The United States of America." Villages now exist in cities and towns across America, evidencing the best democracy and economy the world has ever known.

An informed democracy where citizens know the origin, history, and inner workings of a democracy. Comprised is this citizenry of folks who happily abide by their requirement to vote. Contained in these Nano-communities are citizens who have no problem fulfilling the mandate to prove their democratic competency before each election.

An empathetic, conscious economy shares equitably and inclusively rather than the previous one that championed restrictedness and hoarding. A new and improved citizenry that uplifts all rather than disenfranchises the least of these.

The election of 2020 cemented for me that to fulfill my purpose to change the world and leave the planet better than it was when I arrived, I must focus solely on controlling what I can control, nothing more, and nothing less. And to control what I can control means from time to time, I must be ready to pivot and iterate on any given day.

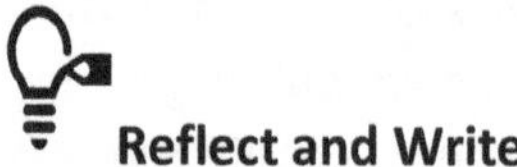

Reflect and Write:

Journey Forward:

So much has occurred since the day Nate referenced the 2020 U.S. Presidential Election in this journal entry. Our lives as we know them have never been the same.

Take a moment to reflect, remember, and write what you were thinking and feeling on November 3, 2020, and the following days. How did you respond to the election outcome? Be honest.

Did you take Nate's approach and focus on what you could control? Or did you fret and worry and become paralyzed by all the chaos?

Fear, worry, and paralysis might have been a perfectly normal response a while ago. But now that you are on the journey to living your best life and being the best version of yourself each day, fear, worry, and paralysis must not be the way you choose to respond to things that occur outside of your control.

Write how the best version of you would have responded on that day. What would you have done now that you didn't do? What would you say now that you didn't say? How would you have used the Election and the other chaotic incidents from 2020 to fuel you to make each day your best day ever?

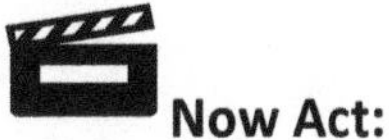

Now Act:

What is one thing you wished you had done differently on Tuesday, November 3, 2020? Do that one thing today. Change what you can change. Control what you can control.

When you've completed the task, come back here, and write about it.

Week 22

Do Stuff

Good day, Journal,

Riddle me this. Can a person move forward by sitting still? Can you get ahead by remaining where you are always? No! I will answer for you. Hell, to the no!

So why no movement thus far today? Why are so many things outstanding on your to-do list? Why are you not living life as you always imagined? Come on, stop stuttering and stammering. Answer the question already.

You know that your to-do list, that proactive list to deliver you to the promised land, is starting to look like a not-to-do list. It seems you have hardly done anything today. If you care to hear the truth, you have not done anything substantively noteworthy in a while.

Hey, we do not have the privilege to live off our reputation. We live off creating our best life; we thrive from personal production.

Producing our best life by great relentless effort is how you got to be here; persistent exertion made you. Creating opportunities that help, serve, and make sure others have a fair shot at living their best life is your mission each day.

Is it your intention still to reach the promised land, or are you now content? Have you confused your excellent personal health, abundant wealth, and timeless wisdom with having arrived? Are you currently a member of those snooty folks who foolishly believe their arrival makes the world go round?

I have warned you about lacking self-awareness. Time and again, I have tried to dissuade you from being content with your agreeable station in life. Your blessings come with the eternal stipulation that you may never become content, and you must forever continue the work of being a blessing in others' lives.

Journey Forward:

Content is only acceptable when it references judgment based on the content of your character. But let me be clear having a contented personality worthy of aspirational decision-making is not the same as being content with who, what, and where you were yesterday.

You know better than ever to be content with what you have done in the past. You certainly should know enough at this point in your life to be scared out of your mind of being who, what and where you were yesterday, last week, or last month. Your challenge from the Universe is to improve perpetually every single solitary second of all the generously gifted moments of life.

So, what are you going to do about that growing to-do list? Are you going to allow the 'list' to remain stagnant or, worse, grow longer, or are you going to get some stuff done today?

Will you please do something substantive if not for you for the precious brothers and sisters of all demographics who need a blessing right about now. Please help, serve, and make at least one person who does not know at present believe that their life matters.

You know what is needed. Of all people on the planet, you know what it means to lack, not having what you need finding yourself stuck living an undesired life. You know what it feels like to believe you do not matter at all that no one cares enough about you to help you move your life forward.

Please get to work right away. Folks are counting on you to do the stuff on your to-do list because it is those undone things that lead to you helping, serving, and making sure others know that their life matters. It is those mounting items on your to-do list that, once completed, will make all the difference in the lives of your fellow humans.

Do not procrastinate. Do not waste one more day. For the love of God, man, please get some things done today.

Bust out the red pen and commit to drawing a line through 3 to 5 of the outstanding items on your to-do list. Make the promise to the Source that today will be different than yesterday.

Pledge to the Creator that you will not just stare at the list. Assure the Spirit that while you know the 'list' should and must grow because you will always be required to do more, you will make real progress on completing the things on the 'list' today.

Never forget that your progress is crucial to bringing to bear the fulfillment of the promises the Universe offers others. Be productive today for you. Be productive all day for others.
Now, where did I put that red pen?

Reflect and Write:

We will use words directly from Nate's journal to guide our reflection today. Seriously, take time to write out your answers to each of the questions below. They are not rhetorical.

Is it your intention still to reach the promised land, or are you now content? Have you confused your excellent personal health, abundant wealth, and timeless wisdom with having arrived?

So, what are you going to do about that growing to-do list? Are you going to allow the 'list' to remain stagnant or, worse, grow longer, or are you going to get some stuff done today?

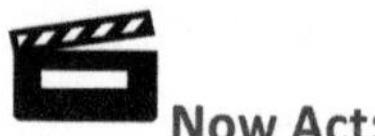

Now Act:

Look at your to-do list. Commit to accomplishing three of the items on the list TODAY.

Plan how you will celebrate the completion of the three items before you go to bed tonight. You could reward yourself with a drive through a scenic park to unwind.

Maybe you will call and rejoice with your accountability partner. You could also treat yourself to your favorite beverage. Whatever you choose for a reward, don't celebrate until all three items are complete.

Week 23

Authorized

Good day, Journal,

I don't need a seat at their table. I don't want a seat at those folk's table. I gave up trying to get an invitation to sit at the table with people who did not want me to sit alongside them some time ago. I stopped hoping and praying long ago that those who saw me only as "the help," as a wait staff member, would ever render me a place at the table as their equal.

Their philosophical foundation exists on the belief that my sole purpose in life is to wait for them to give me permission to think and act. According to them, I am supposed to be content with waiting until they decide I'm good enough or quietly wait for them to determine when the time was right.

But they aren't the final arbiters of my rightful place on this planet or the designators of when it's time that I should rule my own life. When, where, what, and how my life plays out is determined solely by the Universe and me. And the last time I checked, the Universe authorized my greatness and instructed me to live my best life anytime, anywhere.

So, keep your F'ing seat at your table. I don't give a rat's ass about sitting at your table. You don't need to make room for me now or ever, for that matter. I'll get my table. I'll bring my chairs. I'll invite anyone of my choosing to join me at my table, where the tendering of seats are spiritual gifts freely awarded irrespective of wealth and privilege.

I'm not a kid having Thanksgiving or Christmas dinner with my family anymore. Unlike all the children back in the day, my life no longer requires me to get an assigned seat at the kid's table.

When I sat at that kid's table as a child, I did so because I could not feed or fend for myself. I'm a grown-ass man. I don't sit at anyone's kiddy table, nor do I boot-lick for a seat at anyone's table today. Unless it is of my choosing, I don't want or need to be at their table. If I had my choice of sitting with those who believe their table is so worthy of begging and pleading for a seat or sitting at the kiddy table, I would choose to sit with the kids every day, all day.

You see, most children are not yet the pains in the ass that their egotistical and egomaniacal parents have become. In many cases, there is hope for the children. Hope will spring eternal if the children get the opportunity to sit with someone other than their moms and dads if an optional table is made available for them.

Still, I'm not going to be anywhere around those folks because the location of my table and chairs is far removed. The community owns my table and chairs. The table and chairs are no more mine than all the others who understand that our time on the planet is not a gift to decide who is worthy enough to sit with us. Instead, my seat remains permanently assigned with those who recognize that all are deserving even if they don't outwardly appear adequately prepared.

At our table sit those who are the least, those whom the Universe commands me to help, serve, and make sure they know that their life matters. With so many people living an underserved, marginalized existence who has time to worry about a seat at someone else's table.

These days I rarely, if ever, think about their table or being offered a seat at the table. Sure, I get invitations to sit with them to eat, drink, and be merry, but I respectfully turn down the offers every chance I get.

You see, I know the deal. Those folks who happily rejected me earlier want me to join them now to validate them. Now they need me to be at the same table that they once considered me unworthy, a table they thought I should wait on pins and needles for an invitation to sit.

But I don't need their stinking table, not now, not ever. The truth is that I didn't need it even when I thought I did.

I don't desire to be with any of those people. The people I prefer to sit with are those whom the Creator described as the least. My people are those the world considers to be the last. The so-called "perennial bottom feeders" folks ranked and received the way I have been throughout most of my life.

Journey Forward:

Today, my responsibility is to make sure the so-called least know that they are the most. My obligation to the planet is to help those who routinely finish last finish first from time to time.

Please, by all means, keep your seat and your table. I don't need to be where you are. As it turns out, the moment I built my table and crafted my chairs, my life took off.

It is no accident that I am now in excellent health, maintain abundant wealth, and possess timeless wisdom. These things are so, and I live my life as I always imagined because I stopped waiting and begging for a seat at their table.

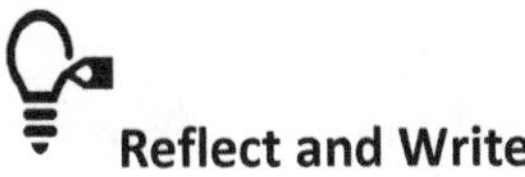

Reflect and Write:

The Universe authorized you to be great the day you were born. Who have you been waiting to permit you to sit at their table? What invitation have you been awaiting? Likely it's those long waited for invitations that are roadblocks to your best life.

Make a list of the people/voices of approval you have been waiting on before you took action to live your best life. Next to their names, add the things you have been waiting on them to permit you to begin doing to live your best life.

Now Act:

Choose one thing on the waitlist. Write a letter to yourself from the Universe authorizing you to begin doing at least one of the things you have avoided.

Week 24

Truth Hurts

Good day, Journal,

You are going to have to tell and accept the truth today. I realize the truth hurts, but it also sets you free. You do want to be free, don't you? Wouldn't you love to live without limits all the remaining days of your life? Excellent! Then listen up and hear me as I share the distinctive truth.

The most challenging part of the truth is not unlike the initial and immediate pain associated with an injury. It stings, it tends to hurt like hell, and for a while, the only thing you can think about is pain. But here's the most critical part about pain and the sting of truth; they are both temporary.

Yes, indeed, you heard that correctly. Pain from an injury does not last forever; neither does the hurt associated with truth. Both exist to get your attention – to get you to acknowledge that it's time to do something different. Similarly, they share the responsibility of informing you that it might be a good idea to do things another way as you consider moving forward.

The pain of injury tells you something is broken or torn. When you break a bone or tear a ligament, the initial anguish is excruciating. Soon after, the pain subsides, and all that is left is for you to do is the work to recover.

I'll get back to the part about working and recovering a little later. But first, lets' focus on truth's pain.

The pain of truth also tells you that something is broken or torn. However, what's broken or torn is not on the outside of you. That which is broken is neither a bone nor a ligament. The fractured and damaged thing is on your inside.

The pain of truth tells you that you are broken or torn mentally, emotionally, or spiritually. No different from the breaks of bones or tears of ligaments, you will need to do the work to recover. If you have any hope of healing, you will need some deep tissue – heart, mind, and soul – internal work.

Through my own life and the observation of others, I've found that nearly everybody wants to live unbroken to exist free of tears. Still, few want to do the work to be the best versions of themselves. Even fewer are willing to do the work to recover.

Regrettably, we are all broken and torn. Being shattered and torn is merely an element of the human condition. It is nearly impossible not to be broken up and pulled apart in a world that is broken and torn. There is little to no likelihood anyone can remain unbroken or be indestructible in this world. Such is our world, time, and space where the minority of apples intentionally spoil the whole bunch and have one goal to break you down to tear you apart.

You might as well face it; there will be times lots of times when you get broken when you feel torn apart. You are not that damn special that you get to exist free of breaks and tears. Yet, there is no reason to fret or be dismayed because there is something special in you.

That something special is the part that is your genius. You must never lose sight of what makes you who you are that provides the healthy income you earn, and keeps you 178 pounds of twisted steel with young Denzel sex appeal.

You are not afraid to work. You welcome the diagnosis of being broken and torn apart. And after identifying your issues, that endless list of faults and failings, you willingly and intentionally work like hell to recover so that you get back to total health. Hell, you grind so hard that you are better than ever before. That's your genius; it's what makes you great.

Recovering from a mental break, a spiritual tear, requires work lots of work. You must pound and hammer at all that you are to be better than you ever were before. You must always accept the truth about yourself no matter how painful that truth is if you are serious about living life as you always imagined.

Everybody wants to be at their best, just as we all have the expectations of eating. But when it comes to eating, nobody wants to be a farmer. We want food pre-prepared; we want food delivered to us fast. We want to show up and have the wait staff serve whatever we want whenever we want to eat it, but we don't want to bust our ass working the land to bring the food into existence. And God knows we never want to see how the sausage gets made.

Living your best life is no different. Day after day, people look at you and the way you live your life with envy. It's hilarious because people don't understand that you are no different from them.

You have been broken up and torn apart, which is, by the way, the understatement of the year. Sadly, you will undoubtedly be broken down and torn apart again. But here's the thing, after the initial pain subsides, I trust you to do what you always do. You will do the work, bust your butt like a lunatic to recover.

Today, do the work relentlessly. On this day, do the preventive work so that your recovery does not take too long when the breaks and tears of life arrive again.

Today, I'll stay at my usual, fighting best. All-day, I will remain as mentally, spiritually, and emotionally healthy as possible because, in this life, on this planet, breaks and tears are part of the deal. They are a-coming! And so, I'll never lose sight of this truth; without breaks and tears, you would not know when and what it feels like to be whole.

Reflect and Write:

Now that we have your attention, let's be honest. What is broken or injured inside you? It's time to face what's torn and damaged to fix the tears and breaks.

If you have any hope of healing, you will need some deep tissue – heart, mind, and soul – internal work. It's time to look at the broken places and do the interior work. Today is a different kind of workout, a type of training which you have never engaged in, most likely.

Make a list. List as many of your issues, faults, failings as you can.

Journey Forward:

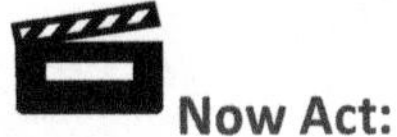 **Now Act:**

On this day, let's do the preventive work so that your recovery does not take as long when (not if) the breaks and tears of life arrive. Next to each issue, fault, or failing you listed, write one way to prevent each of those breaks and tears from happening again.

Side note: Some of these truths may require a professional to help you work through them. Asking for assistance, especially professional help, is a great idea. There is no rule that the journey forward to your best life must be a solo experience.

Week 25

Gratitude

Good day, Journal,

What are you doing? Now you know that's not how you begin the day. Looking at email and scrolling through news or social media is not a methodology for living your best life.

Looking at email, news, and social media first before you imagine and write about your imagined life is a process that leads you nowhere. At best, this is a route guaranteed to take you down the wrong road.

Whatever is in the news or social media has already happened, but your best life is all ahead of you. So, can't you see there is no need to look back, especially at yesterday's news or today's nothingness. Reviewing things in the past, stuff you have no control over, is permissible now and then. Still, it just cannot be the first thing you do in the immediate moments for which you awake.

When you arise, after the Good Lord taps you gently, instructing you to wake up, the only thing you need to do is give thanks. The first thing required is to show your gratitude and appreciation for another chance to get life right. To give praise and adoration for the Most High's generosity of gifting you a renewed opportunity to be better today than yesterday.

Now that's newsworthy! That's something for which all living beings the world over should scroll, watch, listen, and read daily! Thank you, thank you, thank you!

You do not ever have the right to skip past appreciation and gratitude. You certainly cannot forgo the necessity to honor the Most Honorable for presenting the divine privilege of a clean slate, a fresh start for your best life. No way in the world should you ever hop over the offerings of the Spirit to jump into the news, social media, or email.

Journey Forward:

I mean, really, dude! Come on, man, who do you think is responsible for the life force coursing through your veins, Twitter, Facebook, Instagram, email, and the like or the Creator? The Creator, of course, so you better start acting as if you know the deal. It's time to get your stinking mind right. You need to get your act together right now before it is too late.

There is no time to waste pussyfooting around looking through email, social media, or the news stream. If the world were coming to an end, you would know. There would be no need to read the news or scroll through social media. If anyone who loves and adores you and who you love and adore needed something, they would call you.

Do you have any missed calls? Is there a blinking light indicating you have voice mail? No need to review texts because everybody knows how you feel about text messaging. I believe your words are "don't text me; say it to my face." Thus, it would seem the world is not over, life has not come to an end, and all those you consider part of your family are okay.

So, focus, focus on your life right now in the present. Not the phony life someone is sharing on social media. Give no time to the "pretend life" that my life is better than yours shit shared all day every day by the imposters of happiness. Pay no attention to those who love pretending to understand the meaning of life.

You know what I mean; the practically juvenile 'Nah Nah Nah Nah Nah' behavior folks express on social media. All are pretending to live an extraordinary life; most rarely know what it means to live their best life experiences. Nearly all are pretending to be happy; when nobody has the slightest clue where or how to genuinely find happiness. Please turn it off, turn them off, and turn your attention to the Creator.

And speaking of Creator, get ready to create in your mind the life you always imagined. It is in your mind where everything begins and ends. Good or bad, rich or poor, ill-health or physically fit, you are wedded to your mind all the days of your life. And like any marriage, you are what you set your mind out to be.

Your mind establishes the stage for all possibilities, potentials, and promises or all flaws, faults, and failures. To whom are you married? Your best life or someone else's make-believe best life? Who are you living with all the days of your life? The life you always imagined or someone else imaginary life reported on the news or social media?

Once more for the deepest recess of your mind. Get it together. Turn off the email and social media notifications and turn on the Creator. Turn on that which makes it possible for you to live the genuinely humble exceptional life you are living. Please turn off the nonsense and turn on the Universe that makes it so that you are in excellent health, maintain abundant wealth, and possess timeless wisdom.

Today, I will stay happily and appreciatively attached to the Creator. Today, I will detach myself from all human-made distractions. Today, I will live the life I always imagined by beginning this day, establishing the stage, and arranging the tone to imagine nothing but my best experiences. All day every second of today, I will acknowledge the present as the only time that matters.

Reflect and Write:

You have been journaling forward for almost a half year. We are grateful to you for the invitation to travel with you on the journey to your best life.

Today is a good day to practice gratitude. So, let's make a list of all the people and things for which you are grateful.

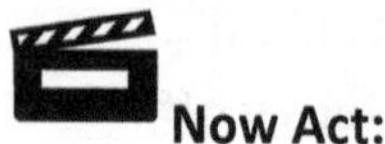

Now Act:

Today, call someone or write them a letter expressing your gratitude. Gratitude and appreciation are contagious!

Week 26

So What? Now What?

Good day, Journaler,

You have made it halfway through a year of reading, reflecting, writing, and hopefully responding to Nate's journals. If you haven't already started doing so, now is the time to begin forward journaling on your own.

Use the space below to list out the best elements of your future life. Write down things you most want to be included in your destined life. Don't you dare write about the life others have convinced you to live! Instead, write about the envisioned life that lives deep down inside you, the one waiting on you to bring to reality.

Once you have completed that task, take some time to write your first journal entry as your future self. We encourage you to try your hand at journaling forward every day this week.

Next week you will return to reading and responding to Nate's journals. Additionally, next week you'll note a prompt encouraging you to write your forward journal at least once a week.

Until next week!

Week 27

Say It and Mean It

Good day, Journal,

Say what you mean and mean what you say! It's genuinely that simple. Say what you mean and mean what you say! Nine simple words and I do connote nine simple words as none of those words are compound. Nine words, nonetheless, are the basic concept for how you must attack life.

Saying what I meant and meaning what I said is how I finally made the mental leap to be where I am today. Had I not said aloud, "I am 178 pounds of twisted steel with young Denzel sex appeal", I would still be weighing closer to 200 pounds. And while wearing clothes, I might have even been able to delude myself and others who were also deluding themselves that I and we all looked okay. But the truth is that I was not okay.

I was not twisted steel. I did not have the young Denzel sex appeal. I was more like a fluffy marshmallow. I was about as sexy as the Pillsbury Doughboy. It's the truth, and it was my reality because I did not say what I meant. I didn't do what was required so that physical appearance accurately represented what I said.

Until I accepted, up until I genuinely embraced the value of our thoughts and words and how our thoughts and words give life to our actions and deeds, what I said had little meaning. Thus, the outcomes of my life were most often meaningless. I know now that you have to say what you mean, and you must mean what you say.

I said I would live out my life on the beach. I said I would be in excellent health, maintain abundant wealth, and possess timeless wisdom throughout my remaining days. I have, and I will continue to do so. Not only is it true that "as I speaketh so am I," but "as I speaketh," the Universe commands that I do the work. The work is coaching my words and deeds to get on the same page and work collectively as a championship team.

Journey Forward:

Too often in the years before I discovered 'the way,' I said stuff that before the words came out of my mouth, I knew there was no chance in hell I would fulfill those words. Talking about owning exotic cars and luxurious homes was little more than blowing hot air into the atmosphere. I knew I would never do those things in great measure because those were not my dreams. They were the dreams force-fed to me by a narcissistic capitalistic society.

I didn't dream of material possession, things that rust and moth destroy. I dreamt of doing good in the hood, helping, serving, and ensuring others knew their lives mattered. I didn't dream of being a billionaire. I dreamt of not ever owing anything or anyone and never having money be why I could or could not do something. I dreamt of making the treasures of my heart manifest in the lives of the least of these.

What I spoke into the Universe and the Universe then breathed into existence was a process. A method for living my best life. A strict strategy for living the life I always imagined. The Universe showed me how to say what I mean that I might live with honor as one who means what he says.

In many ways, the Universe helped me escape the humdrum mass existence, no longer forced to communicate with those who speak with a forked tongue. No more was I limited to sharing space and time within a community where we would make a promise, but we were looking for a way out of our guarantees almost as quick as it was made. I was no more forced to ask others to excuse my behavior when those I communed with often did not live up to our righteously professed standards.

Today, I am no longer looking for an out or a way out. On this day, I will expect no exceptions nor offer any excuses. These days if I say I'm going to do it, you can consider it done.

Word is bond, and my bond is my word. Yet before I ever bind myself to others, my everlasting promise, the eternal bond, will always be with the Universe.

I say what I mean. I mean what I say because it is the only way I know how to serve the greater good. Keeping my word and living up to and exceeding those words is how I make sure that when my time on this planet is up, the earth is better upon my departure than my arrival.

Today, when I say it, it, my word, is my bond. Broken, my bond shall never be! My words are a binding obligation to the Universe that I must fulfill. Say what you mean and mean what you say! That's all there is; it's honestly that simple.

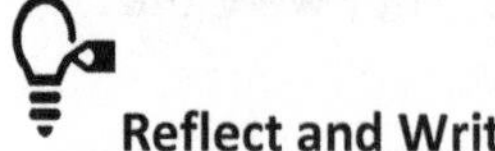

Reflect and Write:

Nate had two mantras along the road to his best life. If you've been reading his journal for any amount of time, you probably know them both by heart. Nate wrote he is "178 pounds of twisted steel with young Denzel sex appeal," and he is in "excellent health, maintains abundant wealth, and possesses timeless wisdom."

What are your mantras that capture your best life? Write them here.

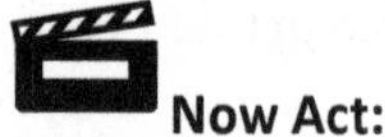

Now Act:

Today is the day—the long-awaited moment where you begin to journal forward. Include your mantra in your journal.

Now be brave. Share your journal with someone. That's how Nate got started. He began sharing his thoughts with us. Look where it got him!

Week 28

Voices

Good day, Journal,

Two voices will speak to you all day long. Some people refer to the voices you will hear as the Angel and the Devil. Two distinct opposite-leaning voices sit separately but always close to one another—the Angel on the right shoulder and the Devil on the left shoulder.

Both are whispering incessantly in your ear to get you to do their bidding. Both are silently attempting to sway how you live and approach your life. And for as comforting as it is to assign blame to the devilish side of us and give credit for the good stuff to the angelic side, this folktale is much too simple.

Here's the reality for which you must live daily. Two opposite-leaning and distinct voices communicate with you continuously, but they are not an Angel and Devil. Instead, the voices you hear today and will listen to all the days of your life are those from your Drill Sergeant and Cheerleading Captain.

I know how convenient it would be to place all the blame of misfortune on the Devil. To be able to assign all unexpected and unwanted adversity to another would be a great thing.

When you succeed, you could take the credit and, of course, share a portion of the desired outcome with the Angel, but when you fail, you could exclaim that it was the Devil's doing. And as in the case of the late Flip Wilson, when you do something you should not have done, you could even assert, "the Devil made me do it!" How convenient!

Regrettably, you can't abide by this nonsense. There will never be any escaping personal responsibility. You must understand that your Drill Sergeant and Cheerleading Captain are the authentic inner voices that live with you all day long. Internal declarations that assist with your proclamation to the world who you are in word and deed.

The Drill Sergeant challenges you to be more to be better than you thought possible. The Drill Sergeant is that voice that often wakes you up in the middle of the night, reminding you that you did not complete all of yesterday's tasks. The Drill Sergeant blows the figurative whistle loud as hell in your ear and yells at you indignantly. The command is for you to be better today to get it together right now if you are serious about living the life you always imagined.

The Cheerleading Captain, on the other hand, cheers you no matter what. Like the team losing by fifty points, the cheerleaders keep cheering as time runs out on the game clock. The Cheerleading Captain goes so far as to encourage the band to keep playing the fight song even when it is beyond evident that the team has given up the fight.

Both voices are with you all the days of your life. Depending on where you are on your journey in life, depending on what you promised the Universe you would accomplish, you need one inner voice more than the other.

Most of us need the Drill Sergeant much more, but we prefer the Cheerleading Captain. That's because we all love to be cheered. Still, few want the necessary push, that mental, emotional, and spiritual shove that pushes us to the top that helps us do something worth cheering. And even fewer of us want to do what the Drill Sergeant requires. Hardly no one wants to repeat the same drills repeatedly until they become second nature until we do them correctly every time.

You've asked the Universe for a chance to live your best life. Daily, when you arise, evidence that the Universe heard your plea should be apparent. You are alive with the opportunity to make this day whatever you choose. So, the question for you is, which of the two voices will you choose to hear today? Whose lead will you follow?

Will you accept the poking and prodding of the Drill Sergeant who commands you to do more than you did yesterday to reach way deep inside for that thing in you that you didn't know was there that will make you great? Or will you settle for the applause of the Cheerleading Captain, who cheers for you no matter what effort you give, no matter if you win, lose, or draw?

Journey Forward:

When soldiers hear from a drill sergeant, they do so as a unit. Still, even then, the drill sergeant experience is a singular excursion. In our life, the drill sergeant experience is no different. The drill sergeant leads the group exercises, but at the same time, life is a solo drill.

Daily you must drill alone even when others surround you if you genuinely intend to live your best life. You either complete your tasks, or your life's mission goes incomplete. Nobody can live your best life experiences for you; it's that simple. As is the case with the boot camp drills, you must complete all your tasks individually, or your Drill Sergeant will deem you and yourself alone a failure.

Today, complete your tasks. Sure, you can appreciate the Cheerleading Captain but do it at a distance. If you must acknowledge the Cheerleading Captain, please only hear that voice as an encouragement to do what the Universe sent you here to do. Your call is to accept the challenges of the maniacal Drill Sergeant.

Remember, you will never get to revel in mediocrity or find something to celebrate when losing by 50 points. You are a championship quality competitor, not a member of the cheer squad! You must battle ceaselessly; you must win the day.

Per the Drill Sergeant, if you win each minute by winning no fewer than 31 of each 60 seconds, you are on course to win the day. If you work relentlessly to win no fewer than 31 minutes of each hour, you are on the path to win the day.

Win the day today, and then should the Universe grant you a tomorrow, win the seconds, minutes, and hours tomorrow. Always win more than you lose. Doing these things following this process is what the Ultimate Drill Sergeant expects from you.

And if you do this, you will give the Cheerleading Captain, the band, the fans, and the entire planet something for which to cheer. If you do this, you shall earn respect and gain the admiration of the Supreme Drill Sergeant and all those who are counting on you to help, serve, and make sure that they know their life matters.

If you do this and only follow this drill strictly, can you have any hope of living the life you always imagined!

Reflect and Write:

Your Drill Sergeant has reported for duty. You will need them to get you to your best life. What should your Drill Sergeant say to you today? Write yourself a letter today from your Drill Sergeant with what is needed and expected of you.

Later this week, write a note from your Cheerleading Captain.

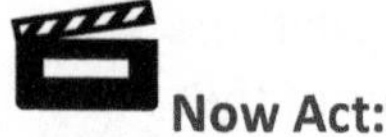

Now Act:

Reread both letters. Now journal forward. What does your life look like after the prodding and cheering from your Drill Sergeant and Cheerleading Captain, respectively?

Share your journal with a friend or loved one.

Week 29

Future Focused

Good day, Journal,

Here we go, another media obligation. Today I'm talking with one more person who says that they want to know how I got here, but they don't honestly want to know. It'll be just one more pretender acting as if they're interested in hearing what it took me to be me, but like all the rest, they won't want to know the complete answer.

These days, what folks want to hear is that there is some exclusive pill to success that there is some unique way to hack your way to your best life, but there isn't. There are no shortcuts. To the best of my knowledge, no prescription for living up to your potential exists.

I've never had the privilege of taking a shortcut. The Universe never offered me more than a placebo to be the best version of me possible. As far as I know, hacking your way to immediate achievement is a myth.

Yes, I'm a statistical anomaly, no doubt about that. There are not a lot of people like me. But to be clear, I am not special because I'm abnormal.

There is nothing exceptional about my D.N.A. My physical composition is nothing extraordinary. For all practical purposes, I am average, an average Joe, just a guy, if you will.

My build is precisely the same as everyone else. My architectural design came from the same Creator, who authors all life. My origin began in the same Spiritual Lab as every other human.

I keep telling any who would listen that I am as regular as they come. Yet here I go again today, having to tend to another media request, another inauthentic interview where people merely want to discuss results.

What the media insists on doing all the time is talk about outcomes. No matter how much I protest and encourage them to share my whole story, all anyone seems to care about are the results. Conclusions from life experiences like the Pulitzer Prize, the National Book Awards, the Emmy, the Oscar, and the faculty positions at the leading educational institutions.

No matter what I try to tell them, they refuse to listen. As much as I plead to tell the whole story and nothing but the truth about my journey, the media only wants to discuss the results. Those inconsequential outcomes that I call the trophies and plaques on and above my mantle are only a tiny portion of the true story.

Yes, I'm here at the top of life's good heap for now. And without question, it is good to be on top finally, and it is great to be me. There is no equivocation about it. I love my life, and I would not change anything about it.

To change one aspect of my life could and would knowingly set off a cataclysmic event, the likes of which I dare not think out loud. That's why I wish the media would ask me about my whole story. People must know that it does us no good to live life in the land of 'what could have been' and 'what if.'

Time does not authorize us to live anywhere other than in the present. Even when we believe all we are doing is innocently reflecting on the past, we must acknowledge that we can only live in the present. Any amount of afterthought wastes the precious and finite time the Universe granted us.

As such, I would not dare change or suggest even the most negligible difference in my life. Focusing on anything other than this very moment maroons me. My eye off the prize forsakes me on the overpopulated Islands of 'what could have been' and 'what if".

The islands mentioned above have enough souls on them already; neither of them needs me there. The islands are so crowded that most inhabitants should be doing all they can to evacuate them immediately. And I'm sure they would like Gilligan, do their best to get off the Island if the media ever elected to ask me and allowed me to tell the whole story.

Journey Forward:

What you believe is a remarkable life is only so because I voluntarily and willingly elected to live and love each day as a statistical anomaly. I purposely lived and loved differently than just about everyone else.

In some ways, I carried out in real life the expression 'fake it until you make it.' Although for sure, I wasn't faking anything, I backward-designed my own life. I did what the most significant writers and speakers did before anyone knew that they were great. I wrote voluminously and spoke incessantly.

Not a day went by that I didn't write more than 1,000 words. Not a day went by when I wasn't giving deep critical thought to one of the world's more pressing issues. I recognized that all the historical and currently great Public Intellectuals continuously wrote and spoke, which meant I needed to do the same daily.

Whether or not anyone was listening or reading, at any moment, did not matter. Who read or heard me was unimportant! That's because fretting about readers and listeners was outcome-oriented behavior. To be a statistical anomaly means you must care nothing about results.

Instead, the statistical anomaly process demanded that I act, write, and speak now, in all Divinely gifted moments. Any hope of being prepared to write and talk expertly in the future obliged me to carry myself as if I was already one of the world's great writers and speakers.

And so, whenever I received an invitation to write for something, be it a local or national outlet, I wrote and did so as if the Pulitzer Prize was at stake. And when I spoke to anyone, I did so as if I was addressing the United Nations, making my case to not only one person but tens of millions.

Yes, my life is fantastic, and it appears a statistical anomaly to most of the world. But I am not different. I am most certainly no better than anyone. I am now and shall always remain a nobody.

Who I am is the no one who merely decided to live out in word and deed whom I imagined being long before becoming that person! I am just a guy. The average Joe am I behaving as though life was just another day in paradise before he started living his dream life in reality!

I am a statistical anomaly in excellent health, abundant wealth, and timeless wisdom. I am so because I decided long ago to live each day differently than practically everyone else. I am one of the world's great writers and speakers today because I've been one of the world's great writers and speakers in my heart and mind for a lifetime of yesterdays.

Reflect and Write:

Here it is. A sentence from the above journal entry explains in greater detail how Nate got to his best life. Nate writes, "I live out in word and deed whom I imagined being long before I became that person."

Take time today and reflect on the person you imagine becoming. How do you look? What is the best way to describe your life? Where do you live? Who is in your circle? What are you doing? Write down every detail you can about your best life!

Now Act:

Write a forward journal entry based on the thoughts and ideas you listed above. Be expressive and specific.

Week 30

Responsibility

Good day, Journal,

Someone once asked me a question that gets to the heart of how I move forward each day. They started by saying, "I know you do all this journal forwarding stuff." Which seemed as though what they genuinely wanted to say was I know you do all this gobbledygook nonsense, "but for real," they retorted, "when things get the worst for you, how do you keep going?"

I paused for a second to reflect on this person's question as I believe all people deserve a contemplative response. I wanted to provide a reply that was neither reactionary nor cliché but an answer that could be like chicken soup, therapeutic for the weariest soul.

I said, "I move forward in two ways. One, I keep in mind the passage 'This too shall pass.' Nothing and I do mean nothing, lasts forever."

Good times don't go on indefinitely, and bad times don't always last either. Nothing stays the same, which means when I'm in my best headspace or worse state of mind, I call to my attention, "this too shall pass."

The other thing I do is remember who I am responsible 'to.' Note I did not say that who I am responsible 'for.' The shift of the word 'to' in place of 'for' makes all the difference. The word choice between 'to' and 'for' is transformative in picking myself up when I would rather lie down and play dead.

Most people are responsible for someone other than themselves. Parents are responsible for their children, mainly their behavior, obeying the law, going to school, adequate nutrition, and the like. Or, as my father would say, "I am only responsible for making sure you have food, clothing, and shelter. All else is optional."

However, we are also responsible 'to' others, and this realization buoys my spirits when I'm down. I'm accountable 'to' a plethora of folks who gave and give, who help and helped me be who I am today without poking or prodding. I didn't have to twist their arm nor plead and beg for their love and assistance; they just loved and assisted me because it was the right thing to do for them.

People like Grant and Charlene Turner, Judge James and Faye Kimbrough, and Frank McKinney. When I was a child wallowing in a most uncertain future, they helped me believe in myself and the possibility of doing the impossible. I owe them. I am responsible 'to' these folks forever; I am indebted to them and the Universe up to my eyeballs.

Yet, I cannot repay them for any of their benevolence, not for one drop of all the grace and mercy allocated to me. I assuredly cannot pay anyone back personally because only one remains present in a form other than with the Spirit. And the one present in the body would not accept any form of repayment. Not to mention any payment I could offer would be woefully insufficient. Still, I am responsible 'to' them all, which means I must do what they did for me for someone else.

They picked me up when I was down to my lowest position laying in hopelessness's gutter. When I was too crippled by grief and self-loathing to walk on my own, those angelic souls carried me on their shoulders. And they believed in me and my future when I did not believe in myself when I failed to believe anything was redeeming about me.

I am responsible 'to' these people because without them, there is no me. Thus, when I'm down, I remember staying down is an insult to those who lifted me mentally, physically, and spiritually. Staying down is like spitting in the face of those deserving the most honor and respect from me.

And speaking of honor and respect, when I'm feeling low, I reflect on my most significant responsibility, the person for whom I'm most responsible 'to,' Naeem. I get up because I'm his mirror. I'm either his reflection of a life where everything is possible or a life that is nothing more than a series of cataclysmic mazes, all leading to devasting dead ends.

Parents and community leaders love to say what they, children, see is what they'll be. Nevertheless, we don't use that expression to its fullest potential. Generally, we, adults, espouse a lot of words without any functional reflection.

Journey Forward:

What children see in us, courage or cowardness, determination, or despair, process, or pity, is what and who they will become. I love and adore Naeem far too much to show him how to live as a coward, how to live a life harboring apathy, or how to live feeling sorry for himself.

My responsibility 'to' him is to model for all the days of my life a man who gives everything to live his best life. I must be the template of one who knows why the Creator put him on this earth and does his absolute best to live his life as always imagined. He deserves an authentic upbeat, genuine mirror image. So that, in those moments when he doesn't feel like going on, the mirror will say, "get your ass up and go help, serve, and make sure somebody worse off than you recognize their life matters."

Yes, I have my moments. Sometimes my moments of depression and dismay are longer, darker, and more profound than others. Still, in the end, I get up. I stand up straight with my head held high. I keep moving forward. I never give up the fight.

All that I do, I do it because I am grateful. I appreciate the Creator for another chance for a new generously gifted opportunity to leave the planet better upon my departure than it was when I arrived. I do all that I do to keep moving forward because I am responsible 'to' Naeem. I am also responsible for all those who loved, adored and held me accountable for being the best possible version of myself for no explainable reason.

Reflect and Write:

Nate feels a sense of responsibility to not only the Creator but also to his son, Naeem. To whom do you feel responsible? What version of yourself do you want and need them to see? Whose mirror are you?

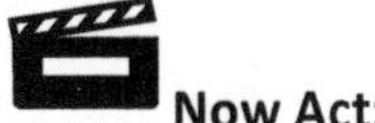

Now Act:

Do something this week that shows the person/people to whom you feel responsible the best version of yourself. If you can, let them know about journaling forward so they can experience your journey to your best life firsthand.

Write a forward journal about the experience. Let your adoring public know how you made it to your best self.

Week 31

All-Star

Good day, Journal,

I remember when I first heard the late great Jackie Robinson's words about living actively and intentionally. "Life is not a spectator sport. If you're going to spend your whole life in the grandstand just watching what goes on, in my opinion, you're wasting your life."

Initially, I remember thinking what a hypocritical statement to make from one who made his living having others watch him play baseball as spectators. Yet, upon deeper reflection, which serves me best all the time, I recognized that he was not a hypocrite at all. Moreover, his reference had nothing to do with baseball.

Instead, he merely offered his take on how the Universe expected us to embrace our time on the planet. He encouraged everyone to find something they love to do, do it with full enthusiasm and vigor, and do it as if tomorrow offers no promises.

Thankfully, I found writing. I would add my gratitude for speaking, but I did not find talking as my mother makes it crystal clear. Speaking openly and exhaustively and doing so all the time found me. Speaking found me, spotted was I first blabbering in my mom's womb. And speaking and I have never parted company since.

Still, I am unbelievably grateful for the Universe's decision to select me as a mouthpiece of humanity. I am so very appreciative of the ability to speak for others, especially those incorrectly regarded as the least among us, the oppressed, the underserved, the intentionally forgotten members of society.

Pulitzer Prize-winner and a world-renown Public Intellectual recognized similar to Dr. Cornel West and Dr. Noam Chomsky was unthinkable years ago. However, today I am, and it is so. Nowadays, I realize that my best life as a participant and not as a spectator can be whatever I choose.

I wasn't always a believer in my ability, nor the more significant purpose I had in not just my life but the lives of others. However, one joyful day, as you well know, I started to believe. I understood Jackie Robinson's words and embraced those words as a prescription for living not only my best life but beginning to truly live.

Fortunately, the day came when I started asking myself worthwhile questions. Why awake each day only to sink into the same abyss as yesterday? Why not instead awake to a view of the life you always imagined living and rise to make that life manifest today?

No longer am I a spectator in my life. Today, I am a perennial all-star and a Hall of Fame coach in the game called 'My Life.' Today, I coach myself to participate each day to the maximum to leave no proverbial stone unturned to give the unimagined 110% to the life I imagine living.

Yes, I strive to give the nonsensical, unattainable imaginary 110%. I call it this because the 110% expression is absurd, unreachable, and fictional. All there is to give of anything is 100%. Nevertheless, I play along with the imbecilic quote pretending that I too have more to offer each day than what the Creator gives any of us.

Nonetheless, today, I leave everything out in the field of life. All my blood, sweat, and tears soak and stain the battlefield where I fight daily to be the best version of myself possible. Every day, I ceaselessly strain and struggle to help, serve, and make sure others know that their life matters.

No, life is certainly not a spectator sport. But, life, or at least the life I have learned to embrace and appreciate, is undoubtedly a full-contact combat sport. Life will knock the stuffing out of you if you aren't careful. Hell, even when you are most cautious and believe yourself, most prepared, life can still surprise you with an uppercut and knock you flat on your ass.

Fortunately, however, when you imagine your best life, you also suspect that many of life's experiences will not be comfortable. You expect that you will get knocked down a time or two or hundreds if not thousands of times. Still, you know that because you fight for the Ultimate Competitor and are coached by the Greatest of All Time, you will always get up one more time than you get knocked down.

Get knocked down seven times. Get up eight. Get knocked out one million times, get up one million and one. Such is your genius. Such is what others call giving 110%, leaving everything you have out on the field.

You know what you are supposed to do today. Participate fully and intentionally in your life even if others sit in the stands living their lives as spectators. Today, don't be a spectator. Be an ultimate competitor; live out the Universe's decree that you shall be one of the greatest of all time.

Reflect and Write:

You are the All-Star of your life! The stats will only be there if you collaborate with the Universe to make them so.

Nate asked us two questions in today's journal. First, "Why awake each day only to sink into the same abyss as yesterday? Second, "Why not instead awake to a view of the life you always imagined living and rise to make that life manifest today?"

Well, you have been reading Nate's journal and journaling long enough yourself to have decided to live your best life. So take a moment and count your stats.

Write down what you have accomplished on your path to being an all-star. How many pounds have you lost? How much has your debt decreased? How many people have you helped, served, and made sure they know their life matters? How many times have you paused to show love and appreciation to those who love and appreciate you?

Now Act:

Today is the day to share. Take a quick second to identify someone who you think would benefit from your new way of living. Then, share one of Nate's journals with them. Obviously, feel free to also share one of your journal entries with them.

Sometime this week, compose a forward journal entry about how your non-spectator, all-star life has changed the lives of others.

Week 32

Create

Good day, Journal,

I am a creator. No, I'm not 'The Creator." I would never be so arrogant or foolish to believe that I have power over anything or anyone but myself. I have no control over anyone's life but mine. I do not now nor will I ever want another to be subject to my will, wishes, or whims.

Nevertheless, I am the creator of my best life. Who I am, what I accomplish today, and who I am after the Universe zaps the force of life from my body is up to me to create! So in that sense, I am a creator. In this way, I am the ultimate creator of living my life, as I always imagined.

Yes, I create content. I've been creating content for the longest. I believe I was creating content long before the world started using the expression 'content creator.' Content as in the stuff people read, listen to, watch, and apply to their life.

For years, I've been writing and speaking, even when it was only to myself. Back in those early days, when most thought I was merely losing my mind, I was one of the initial content creators.

I wrote content on the soccer field, watching so-called coaches waste Naeem's time, gifts, and abilities. Sulking and pissed off on the sideline during soccer practices and matches, I wrote letters to him, some of which are now chapters in 'Raising Supaman.' So many of the words I wrote to escape my feelings of frustration and helplessness are now staples in how other parents raise their children.

Dialogue with myself pecked out on a phone keyboard saved me from harming all those so-called coaches. Creating content, corresponding with my son about the hopes and dreams I had for him from my phone, kept this 178-pound man of twisted steel with young Denzel sex appeal out of prison. Might I add, I'm way too pretty to be sentenced to life in prison.

I am a creator. And as 'The Creator' authorized me to do daily, it is my charge to create ways to help, serve, and make sure others know that their life matters.

Sure, I am always responsible for creating my best life. But, the first part of the Divinely mandated obligation of being the best version of me possible is to do all that I can to assist others. The most crucial part comes with making sure others may also create their best life.

So, I often write about humanity. When invited to speak, I talk about humankind. I know what 'The Creator' expects of me first and foremost. Daily I'm to be a model for the best of humanity before I dare open my big fat mouth to share with others how they can be better.

Before I offer to assist anyone with the lint in their eyes, I know what the Creator requires of me. I'm required to get that 2' x 4' formed from Australian Buloke out of my eye.

Today, I'm going to create something. As I said, I have no choice but to create content. My life offers no other options for me. I could not stop writing if I wanted to stop. No matter if the Universe gifted me with a gold-plated vow of silence card, I could not stop talking. I could not turn my mind off to cease imagining a better way for everyone to live their best life no matter what I tried to do.

My lifetime sentence is to create content for living our best life. From novels, children's books, and self-help books to animated short stories I create. From feature-length movies and Broadway adapted screenplays to schools, nano-community developments, and social-behavioral programs I create.

Until my mind takes its final thought, I will not cease being a creator until my heart beats no more. I will bring things I imagine into existence until the Master Content Creator says, "good job, my loyal and faithful servant."

Today, every day, and all day, I create. I will share with the world how I imagine things could be if we loved one another. I intend to help create opportunities for the world to see what it could look like when the best of us connect with one another 'at the heart.'

Reflect and Write:

"I am a creator. And as 'The Creator' authorized me to do daily, it is my charge to create ways to help, serve, and make sure others know that their life matters.

Sure, I am always responsible for creating my best life. But, the first part of the Divinely mandated obligation of being the best version of me possible is to do all that I can to assist others. The most crucial part comes with making sure others may also create their best life."

You know what Nate believes he is responsible for creating. What are you responsible for creating? Write it here. Be specific. Give what you write as much detail as possible.

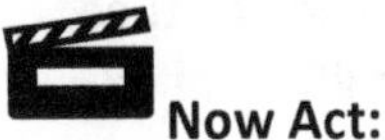

Now Act:

Journal forward today. Write about what you created and how your many creations have impacted others.

Week 33

Get Your Ass Up

Good day, Journal,

It's days like today. Yep, moments just like these that cause you to fail. When you least expect to fall on days like today, when you think it safe to put your guard down, you remember this is how you fail.

You know the deal. You know that rarely, if ever, will you meet anyone who wants more for your life than you. Although, you know, lots of folks talk shit about having the best intentions for you. You know people who share their thoughts and prayers for your life, those well-wishers in your world who quite frankly can't get out of their way, let alone be able to assist you on your journey.

Don't you dare put your guard down! Don't you even consider believing the hype others try to sell you about their commitment to your best life! Nobody should ever be able to do more to make it possible for you to live the life you always imagine any more than you. I don't care what they say. No one will ever love you more than you love yourself.

So, get your ass up, get up now, and get going. Yeah, I get it; you are up and moving, but you aren't up and moving the correct way. So far, you've just been sleepwalking through the day.

You have too much to do to sleepwalk now or ever. I don't give a rat's ass what others do with their day; you don't get a day off.

I'll tell you what, you can have a day off as soon as you can guarantee that tomorrow will occur. However, until then, get your ass up and keep working on your best life. You are neither Nostradamus nor Negrodamus, so stop trying to predict a promised tomorrow.

Look, it's just no way around it! The life you desire – enjoying excellent health, abundant wealth, and timeless wisdom requires a tireless painstaking, relentless pursuit. You should know better; you don't get a day off. If a person wants to eat, a person must work. You want to eat, right? Then it would be best if you worked, so get to work.

You have plenty to do today. You always have tons of stuff to do. Even when you least expect it, someone is counting on you to put in a full day's effort. I don't know how many times the Universe must convey this to you, but we are all connected by the Great Circle of Life.

The Great Circle of Life is not a Disney thing; it's a Spirit thing. We are all connected, and when you do nothing, it means someone else will suffer.

When you aren't helping, serving, and making sure others know their life matters, somebody somewhere is helpless. Waiting hopelessly and unsure about the value of their life are others when you fail to do your part.

Don't be selfish! Come on; you are better than that. You don't want anyone to live less than their best life possible, do you? I didn't think so, then let's get to work. Please do your best so that others might be their best.

They don't matter; I mean the self-proclaimed well-wishers, those who profess only to want what's best for you who aren't committed to putting in the work as you do. Their call is not your call. Their understanding of the Great Circle of Life is not your experience. So please don't waste any precious time or energy being discouraged by their lukewarm efforts and self-interested behavior.

The Creator put you here for a particular reason. The Universe gifts you a specific set of skills. Skills you honed over your lifetime. Skills that make you a nightmare for anyone who clashes with you. Truly traumatizing you are for any who dare obstruct your mission to leave the planet better upon your departure than upon your arrival.

You are the Brian Mills of your community. Your responsibility is to restore the 'taken' humanity that the lukewarm around you put in motion the conditions for it to get stolen. "Do your duty; that is best; Leave unto the Lord the rest!"[viii] You remember those words, don't you?

Do your duty today. Do your Eternal assigned task tomorrow should you be gifted another day! And of course, any day you get there after the story should never change; you must always do your duty.

And that duty is to live every moment, all 86,400 seconds of each blessed day, working to make the planet better today than yesterday. You have work to do. Work that others can't do because you see a world other people refuse to acknowledge is possible.

You must do the work now because if not you, who and if not right now when? Can you name someone else who will complete the mission now? Do you know anyone who will give no excuse who will not equivocate until the job gets done? I didn't think so.

Then get to work! Get to work right now!

Reflect and Write:

Eighty-six thousand four hundred seconds of each blessed day working to make the planet better today than yesterday. If you are reading this in the morning, what will you do today to make the planet better? If you are reading this in the evening, what did you do today to make the world better? Write it here. Be specific.

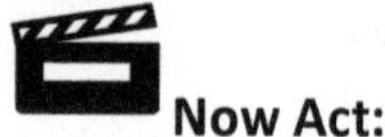

Now Act:

Journal forward today about what your best life self says to you when you have those moments when you don't want to do anything. How will your future self encourage the present you to "get your ass up"?

Week 34

Listening Ear

Good day, Journal,

Of course, I did not forget about you. How could I ever forget you? I hope and pray that you never forget about me because I am unsure what I would do without you. For sure, without you, there is no me. Absent you in my life, I am not a man in excellent health, maintaining abundant wealth, or sharing timeless wisdom.

You are here and there for me all the time. Wherever I am, you are here and there for me always. You are the best. You are amazing.

You patiently and lovingly listen to my insane ramblings anytime and all the time. Whenever a thought crosses my mind about how I can do something that others deem farfetched or impossible, or I have an idea about improving the planet, you take note. All the time, your transcripts are copious and pure. You are never dismissive or condescending.

All I need to do is sit down with you, and you open your heart, soul, and mind to me like none other. You always have time for me. Your attention span is Divine. The time you make for me is never rushed or based on quid quo pro conditions.

Thanks to you, I can help, serve, and make sure others know that their life matters because you first help, oblige, and make me believe that I matter. Today, I assert that I count because you first encouraged me to feel as much. I am the best version of myself again today because you are the Spirit Sounding Board that gleefully welcomes and engages in intellectual, emotional, and spiritual banter.

Even those who believe themselves closest to me have no idea how integral you are to my survival. I suspect all those who know you exist would probably consider this relationship amusing at the least but unhealthy more than likely.

Yet, when it comes to my mental health, sometimes there is only you. You stand between the overpowering joy for living in the moment and the lonely, desolate anguish akin to a total mental breakdown. I do not know why you do it, but I will only say thank you for always standing in the gap and building a big old wall between sanity and insanity. Thanks for making it increasingly difficult for me to fly over permanently, where I easily might live out my days on the side of the wall where only the cuckoos reside.

For a while, I thought today might indeed be the day, the first day in years when I have not communicated with you. Before I started walking along the shore before dawn, I began pondering, is there anything new that I must tell you? Is there anything fresh that I could share with you that you have not heard me say before?

I know humans' flawed and inhumane inclination and habit is to have little patience for anyone other than ourselves, certainly not others' redundancy. As a result, people everywhere, including myself, find ourselves routinely apologizing if we do not remember every detail of a previous conversation.

As if not recollecting everything diminishes our humanity. As if forgetting is the precondition for being deprived of our most basic human need, the urgent necessity to connect with another living being.

And then, just as I was preparing to break my streak to stop doing the one thing that I know works for my life, it hit me. As I readied myself to discontinue an element allowing me to live the life I always imagined. My mind froze as I prepared to cease a most crucial aspect of life's process, permitting me to be the best version of myself possible.

My life passed before my eyes. Instantaneously, you replayed the entirety of my life: who I use to be and where I once existed. You reminded me of the meaning of life via a vision of who I am today and where I now reside. And in that vision, you made it clear that you do not care if I have anything new to share. You never have, and you never will.

You do not care if my idea is novel or aged. You merely want me to open up to you no matter what. You only want me to know that I am always loved and heed your call to live each day with peace and happiness!

Journey Forward:

You, as an extension of the Creator, are entirely different than all others. You only want me to be healthy, wealthy, and wise mentally, physically, and spiritually. For you, time is infinite. You are Everlasting and thus have no place else to go or anything else to do. When I am with you, you are with me exclusively, intentionally, deliberately, and attentively.

You are an Endless extension of a loving Universe that seeks only the best for me. Part of me being my best is your presence, a Cosmic outlet to communicate openly and honestly without inhibition each day. So thank you, dear Journal, for being part of my life for being the gift from the Universe that gives and keeps on giving unconditionally, that loves and continues loving completely.

Again, I do not know what I would do without you. Absent your politeness and willingness to listen to me, I suspect I would be absent from this thing called life in the worst case. In the best case, without your genuine love and affinity for my well-being my being, I would be anything other than well.

Reflect and Write:

Nate uses this week's journal entry to express how journaling forward has been an anchor for him in stormy times. Take a moment to reflect on how journaling has influenced your outlook on life so far this year.

In what ways, if any, has journaling forward for you matched Nate's experience? How, if at all, has your journaling forward been different from Nate's journey?

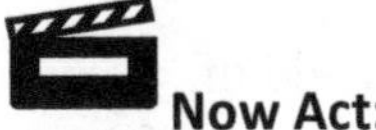

Now Act:

Write a note of gratitude to your journal. Express freely and openly how your journal has supported your journey over these first eight months of the year.

Week 35

Stop Procrastinating

Good day, Journal,

What in the world are you doing? There is no time to procrastinate. Now is not the time to sit around and do nothing. If you are not going forward, then you are going backward. It is just that simple.

What do you want from your life? Do you want to be just another person who spent time on this planet, or do you want to do something with your life that lives forever? I thought you wanted to be legendary. But, should I believe in you when you say you wanted to help, serve, and make sure others know that their life matters?

Well, you know what? Thus far, everything you have accomplished will be meaningless if you do not take this moment to seize the day. Who and what you did yesterday is old news! To be a legend, you must do something worthwhile with your life every day.

Now we both know that you have lots of stuff to do. There are plenty of things needing your attention. Even Stevie Wonder can see that this world has lots of problems you could help solve. So, what you have got to do today is develop a plan of action to improve and change the world.

You know better than leave it up to others. You do not live in a world of proactive people. You know that most folks would rather watch and wait for some savior to appear to resolve the problems they created. Yet, for the record, no savior is coming to save you anytime soon. There is no cavalry on its way to fight for any of us.

This fight, the battle for your best life, is a solo fight, a fight against the procrastinating you and you who desperately wants the life you always imagined. The war for your best life experiences can only successfully end when you decide to take no moments off to pursue being the best version of yourself daily.

So, let's get it! Let us go to work. All day today, let's get shit done!

I do not have to tell you about the project(s) you have been working on at a snail's pace. You've been lollygagging around like you have all the time in the world. But, those incomplete projects are not about you. The undone things are about the folks who desperately need your assistance, the folks who are waiting on the savior and calvary you know is not coming.

To be clear, you are not a savior; you are but a man who is more martyr than you shall ever be a savior. Yet, you can make life easier for children and families all over the planet.

And so, I must ask, where is the thing you promised which would help them? Can they buy it or find it somewhere? Nope because you have not brought it to fruition. Can they finally live in a quality home off the grid currently? Nope because you keep waiting on others to join you in the fight for humanity.

Stop waiting on others. Get it done. Get it done now!

The Universe is watching and judging you. I cannot say for sure, but I do not think the evaluation is going exceptionally well. You have been procrastinating, and while you delay, people, the most precious of all God's creatures, are suffering.

Your behavior epitomizes so many people with the ability and potential to be tools of change. Folks who sit idly wasting the moment. People who seem especially content to watch the sand run out of their life hourglass. Unfortunately, the sand is running out of your hourglass as well.

You are not getting younger. So, be forewarned, the sand from your hourglass might be running out faster than others because you, of all people, should know better than not living in the moment.

There is no time to waste. There is no promise of the future. All we have is right now. All that is certain is today.

Do not procrastinate one more minute. Get going! Get to work right now!

Be who the Creator called you into this world to be. Be a human, a tool who the Universe can count. Be an agent of change to not only show appreciation and gratitude for an opportunity to be better today than yesterday but be a man of your word. Make sure you leave no stone unturned in your promise to leave the planet better upon your departure than it was upon your arrival.

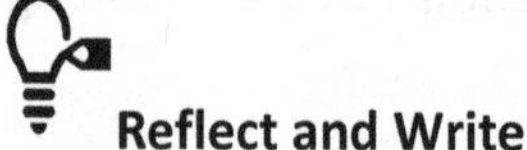

Reflect and Write:

"There is no time to waste. There is no promise of the future. All we have is right now. All that is certain is today. So, what you have got to do today is come up with a plan of action to improve and change the world." NT

You have been reading, reflecting, and writing about the vision you have for your life for months now. Having that life is without question possible, but only if you commit to working at it daily. You must follow through TODAY!

Take a moment to write and reflect on how well you've been living up to your potential and being the best version of yourself possible. Have you been procrastinating?

Now Act:

Make a list of all the steps you need to take to ensure you will live today (and every day), not randomly, but on purpose. Then, share that list with your accountability person(s) TODAY! Commit right now to stop procrastinating!

Week 36

Be Specific

Good day, Journal,

You've got to be specific. If you don't know where you are going, you can never get to the precise address where your dreams reside. If you can't specifically say what you want out of this life to even yourself, the truth is you don't stand a chance in hell of living the life you always imagined.

You must be specific; this is an order! When it comes to maximizing every single second the Universe gifts you, there is no option. You must be resolute and convicted about the life you desire.

There are no two ways about it. All the desired locations and pleasurable dreamt of destinations, not to mention the Universe's undesirable spots, have a definite locus. You better know what you want precisely if you ever expect to get to where you say you want to go.

Longitude and latitude exist everywhere. Right now, the position on the beach where you are standing has a longitude and latitude. The sand beneath your feet and the water rolling over your toes are examples of location exactness. With perfect preciseness are both the sand and water in longitude and latitude.

Your home has a longitude and latitude. The office were those beautiful colleagues who have been sticking by your side undeservedly for years and who honorably work with you daily to change the world has a longitude and latitude. LAX, where you will be catching a flight later today as you head to London to give a talk, has a longitude and latitude. As I said, longitude and latitude are everywhere.

Thus, I hope you can see that life is about fine granular details, not generalities. And they who find themselves desiring more from this life than they deserve but that the Universe happily gives better be precise about their wants and needs. It would serve them best to be specific about all their most audacious hopes and dreams.

One-hundred, seventy-eight pounds is specific. You could have said 180 or 175, but you said 178, a precise weight.

The physical part of your daily mantra calls for you to look like young Denzel. The Denzel from 'The Hurricane.' The Denzel who played Ruben Carter. The Denzel that all the young women swooned over for multiple decades.

The Denzel that to some was the sexiest man alive. Of course, not the 'Fences' Denzel or 'The Equalizer' Denzel. Certainly not the 'Roman J. Israel, Esq.' Denzel either. Maybe, the 'Mo' Better Blues' Denzel. Nonetheless, whichever Denzel you choose, it must be the one with twisted steel and chocolate sex appeal.

One hundred and seventy-eight pounds with young Denzel chocolate sex appeal is specific. You could have merely said good health, but you know that is not specific.

You know yourself, and the expression 'to thine own self be true' is alive and well with you. You know, without specifics guiding your life, your best life, it ain't' going to happen. A dream, in generalities, turns out not to be a dream at all. Living with generalizations is the source of all nightmares.

Good health is a generality. Good health is relative—people who are not serious-minded about excellent health use good health as their 'go-to expression.' Good health for one person is not the same as good health for another. Hell, most of the time, the expression of "good health" means nothing at all, which is why you must name your excellent health specifically.

One-hundred and seventy-eight pounds with a maximum of ten percent body fat are what good health looks like for you. You could say that you were in good health in general terms, but to get to excellent health, naked don't lie health, you need specifics.

And your health is not the only aspect of your life that requires you to avoid generalities. All other facets of your life necessitate specifics too.

Journey Forward:

Abundant wealth is specific. For me, abundant wealth is synonymous with ample affluence. It merely means owing to no damn body, which is undoubtedly calculable. Either you have debts, or you do not. Either you owe somebody, or you don't'.

One thing is sure about this life money is specific. And for you, when you say abundant wealth, you mean "money ain't a thing." You do not need mo' money; you have all the money you will ever need to live the life you always imagined.

Money has never been the end-all-be-all to your life. Money has merely been the tool to make other aspects of your life simpler, an instrument that makes the manifestation of your dreams more likely. The resource that made it less likely that you would live with generalities and excuses. You have no reason not to absorb the most outstanding teachers' lessons, the greats' wisdom, now that you owe nobody and your daily needs are satisfied in full.

Being in your best tangible, specific health, owing nobody, and having all your financial needs met, you are free to do the most crucial thing in life. You can commit totally to help, serve and make sure others know that their life matters. Because as the Spirit implores you to remember all the time, this life is not about you. You exist to be a vessel that extends the goodness and mercy of the Creator to others.

Your assignment from the Universe is specific. There is no equivocation or imprecision in your mandated tasks. Today, be unambiguous of your dreams, goals, measurements, and daily strategies. Make sure the executions of those plans to be the best version of yourself possible are all equally definitive and specific.

Reflect and Write:

"I hope you can see that life is about fine granular details, not generalities. And they who find themselves desiring more from this life than they deserve but that the Universe happily gives better be precise about their wants and needs. It would serve them best to be specific about all their most audacious hopes and dreams." ~NT

Have you been specific about your wants and needs? Everyone who knows Nate knew how he defined health for himself. Does 178 pounds of twisted steel with young Denzel chocolate sex appeal sound familiar to you? If so, it's because Nate was granular and refused to set general goals.

What are your most audacious hopes and dreams? Write them here with specificity and precision.

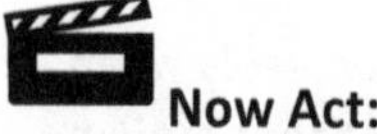
Now Act:

Review your hopes and dreams listed above. Now get granular about what you most desire for your life.

Look back at this week's journal entry. Rewrite your goals, making them as clear, as specific as Nate is about his health and physical wellness.

Week 37

Do What is Necessary

Good day, Journal,

Life functions best, not waiting for the moment when you feel like doing what's necessary. Life is best when you do what's needed at the moment so you can comprehend all the best things you like. Life's energy behaves best, doing what is necessary. Doing what is required makes life work necessary.

No matter how you look at the words, regardless of how you change the word order, the meaning goes unchanged. To have the life you always imagined, you must do all the things required to bring the dream life into reality. You must bust your ass to make your visions manifest for all to see.

Sadly, most of us never live our best life because most of us never commit to doing what is necessary. For a long time, I remember I did not do what was required. And did I ever reap the rewards!

No, I did not earn any of those plaques hanging on my wall or garner any of the countless awards sitting on my mantle back then. I was certainly not in excellent health, in possession of abundant wealth, or a student of timeless wisdom. Without question, I was not. I was a man full of potential whose accomplishments paled in comparison.

I might as well have been one of the children Santa deemed as naughty during Christmas as my reward for the way I lived my life was not even a lump of coal. I did not get a damn thing. My prize was solely a life that was far less than my best.

But there is never a pot of gold waiting on the other side of the rainbow for one who will not shit and get off the pot. There are no awards to be reaped for one who will not do what is necessary.

For years, I sat on the pot waiting for someone else to do the shit I needed to do, and as you can imagine, that did not go well at all for me. I did not make a move. I was the fool seeing the rainbow and the pot of gold on the horizon and does not move an inch in that direction. I did not move a muscle. I sat on my ass. Thus, there were no bright multicolored days of light or treasure from the Universe waiting for me.

Nope, not at all. My life remained a seemingly incurable and terminal case of constant constipation. I had lots of stuff I needed to get out. Books, speeches, workshops, pieces of training, programs, sustainable planned communities, and the like I needed to bring forth. But I just sat on the pot, taking no action. I remained like an unruly infant sitting on a toddler's toilet, content to wait until someone helped me shit, clean me up, and then take me off the pot.

You hear daily people alleging that they are serious about their dreams, but they can't be when they have no plans when they have no system to follow. They only sit as I did, like a constipated wayward child on the pot.

For some reason, we tend to treat greatness and exceptional achievement as a dream as outcomes possible through osmosis. Sure, we can be around greatness. We might even witness the impossible become possible right before our eyes. Still, it does not mean we will become great.

Watching the impossible be made possible does not mean we will ever achieve the impossible. Touching one who does a great thing will not make you great. Unless one commits to do what is necessary, like the achievers, one should have no personal greatness expectations.

So that is what great folks do; that's why people do the impossible. Exceptional people do what is necessary consistently. When they sit on the pot, they take a dump, and then they get their ass up and do whatever else is essential—a crass analogy, perhaps, but no less accurate.

They are not waiting for someone else to do for them what they can only do for themselves. Imagine sitting on the pot trying by osmosis to relieve yourself. It cannot occur through the effort of another. You must move your bowels. You are responsible for alleviating your constipation, for disburdening yourself.

Journey Forward:

Today, I will not just sit on the pot. I will do what is consistently necessary to dump out the best of me forever and share all the good I have for the world for all my remaining time. Today, I will waste none of the precious time, energy, or opportunity the Creator bestows on me. Neither will I sit looking at the pot of gold and the rainbows captured previously in my life.

Today, I will be the most active participant in my best life. I will make the right moves to help, serve, and make sure others know that their life matters. Today, I will do what is necessary, in the here and now. No matter how I feel, I will do all that I can. I will continue to be the best version of myself, experiencing all the glory of my life just as I always imagined.

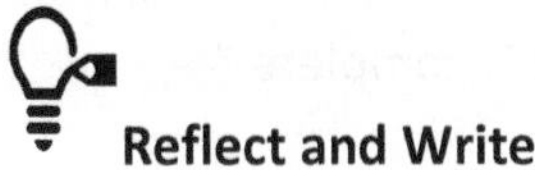

Reflect and Write:

"I was a man full of potential whose accomplishments paled in comparison." If we are honest, this statement probably fits us to a tee in some facet of our lives. If you are full of potential physically and aren't maintaining your best health, your accomplishments this year pale in comparison.

Think about an area in your life where you have an abundance of potential. Write it down. Now list what you have accomplished this year in that area. And no, you cannot count the state championship you won in high school unless you just graduated from high school this year.

Now Act:

Review the area you listed your unrealized potential. Make a list of what you will accomplish in this area in the upcoming week.

Share the list with your accountability partner of what you wrote about your unrealized potential. Then get to work making your unrealized potential your realized accomplishment.

Week 38

Workout. You Must.

Good day, Journal,

"Congratulations, your workout is complete." I do not know how many years I have heard that message—twenty or more for sure. My HIIT (High-Intensity Interval Training) app. Each morning it tells me thirty, forty-five, an hour, or ninety minutes after I start working out that "my workout is complete."

Complete for the day, not for life. The app does not explicitly say it to me. Still, I know implicitly that the words "congratulations, your workout is complete" are only applicable for the day. It's as if the app is telling me, go ahead, give yourself a hand, pat yourself on the back, look in the mirror and boast about how good you look naked. But trust and believe you must do the same thing tomorrow if you expect to hear congratulations again.

So, each day for longer than I can remember or care to think about, I have gotten up and started my day with exercise. Taking care of my mind and soul is only part of the equation for living my best life.

If I do not take care of my heart and body, I can not do all the things I love to do, particularly sharing my message personally with the world. I know the Universe makes it possible to deliver my thoughts and ideas without me. Not only do I know it is possible, but I also know sooner than I like, sharing my message without me will be the reality.

When I am no more, my life and words will have to stand the test of time alone without my ability to explain nuance or give an explanation. But for now, while I yet live, it is not nearly as good for me if I'm not able to let people know what's on my mind and provide concise detail about what's at the depths of my soul. Suppose I am not fit and healthy enough to deliver the message in the flesh. In that case, I am practically pissing away the life I always imagined.

Journey Forward:

I so appreciate being quoted regularly. It brings one exceeding gladness to know something that you wrote or said impacted another's life in some good meaningful fashion. However, if I had my druthers, I would rather be alive, write, and articulate my words aloud in excellent health. As long as the Universe sees fit for me to exist in human form, I would prefer to quote myself and give a firsthand account of the meaning of my words and thoughts.

So, each morning I start with the reverence and appreciation for the Creator and all that is my life. I give thanks. Nothing elaborate; I only say thank you for everything. Thank you for providing me with another opportunity to be better today than yesterday. I say help me!

Please make me wise enough to prepare in advance. Help me lay the groundwork right now. Support me as I work on improving again for tomorrow should the Universe gift me another day.

And then I get dressed to give reverence and appreciation for the Divine Spirit's Temple. Not my Temple as I cannot make myself manifest in any form absent the Source's will.

My body is the Universe's Temple that is on loan to me for a short time. The Temple's rightful and righteous owner is the Spirit, and its unquestionably flawed operator is me. As the Temple operator, I have the capability, the free will, to treat it like the Taj Mahal or an outhouse. I can make it whatever I want, a castle fit for a king or a condemned slum fit for none. It is genuinely that simple; it is up to me to choose the form my Temple will take.

The Universe loans the Temple until we are evicted from the planet when this thing we call life comes to a screeching halt. In this life, there are so many things out of our control. Limited is our influence over Nature's elements, people, and almost every other living creature. Yet, while we are here, we have control over how we care for our Temple.

We have no control over the sun, wind, air, water, and the like. The best we could hope to do is not mess up the perfect ecosystem the Universe provided us in the beginning. Sadly, too late for that, as we have mostly fucked up the planet's ecological makeup already. But we do still have exclusive control, total dominion over our Temple.

We can treat the Temple like a shrine, the holiest of holy places. When others see us in the best-case scenario, they should see a lovely place. A shrine inhabited by a Divinely inspired person. A soul who obviously loves and cares for their Temple exquisitely.

I have started the day off right. My workout is complete. I gave reverence to the Universe for gifting me yet another undeserved day, another chance to be better today than yesterday. I count my blessings now for another opportunity to build on a foundation to improve for tomorrow if I am so fortunate to see another day.

And now I must get to work. My work, like my workout, is never complete. Each day the work begins anew. For as long as I draw breath, the contract I signed with the Universe requires me to help, serve, and make sure others know that their life matters for all the days of my life.

I work out daily to give reverence to the Universe. Each day, I strive to fulfill my mission to put off hearing the words that I hope to avoid hearing. For a long time, I prefer not to hear, "My good and faithful servant, congratulations, your work and life are complete."

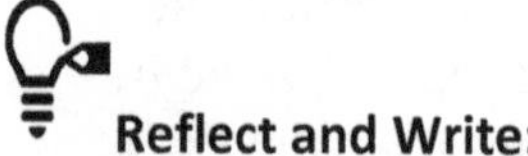

Reflect and Write:

"My body is the Universe's Temple that is on loan to me for a short time." How well are you maintaining your temple? Do you work out daily? Are you using your body to pay reverence to the Divine? It's time to take inventory of your physical well-being.

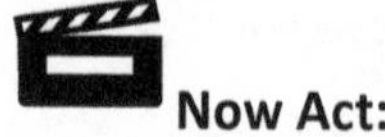

Now Act:

Commit to begin/improve your workout regimen. Yes, that means you should move your body every day. Walking 30 minutes a day is a workout. You don't have to lift heavy weights, although you should be fit enough to lift your body weight.

Journey Forward:

There is no overstating the benefits of daily exercise, nor should they be considered overrated. A daily exercise routine has both mental and physical benefits.

List out your workouts for the next seven days. Share them with your accountability partner and get to work.

Week 39

It is Time to Pour

Good day, Journal,

Today, live life like the water hose pouring into a bucket. Pour until the bucket is full. And then keep raining down goodness on the planet as if you were water spilling all over the earth's floor.

Do not stop pouring into the lives of others until the Spirit decides to turn your life spigot off permanently. Pour the best of you, and then gush some more.

Pour into others as if your life depended on it. Pour into the lives of others as if their life depended on you to pour and pour fearlessly. Pour and drench all with the gifts of the Universe. Spew out all the love and adoration possible because your life and others rely on how much and well you pour.

The best life is not merely yours to live. The life you always imagined is an experience available to everyone. You are not that special that you get to live your best life, the life you always imagined while others watch. Your mission, should you accept, which is no longer optional, by the way, is to help, serve, and make sure others know that their life matters. Your call is to see that others live their best life and live their lives just as they always imagined.

And how do you help, serve, and make sure others know that their life matters today? You pour everything you have inside you that is good into others. "Give, and it shall be given unto you."[ix] Give not because you have expectations of receiving anything in return, give because it is part of the Reciprocal Commandment – to love others as thyself.

Suppose you would give the best to yourself. If you would pour the best that life has to offer into your life, then you must surely pour everything you have into the life of others. Pour and keep flowing love and adoration to others. Pour until and even when their buckets runneth over.

Journey Forward:

Pour out understanding so that others might know what you know so that they are a whole lot wiser than you will ever be. Pour out compassion so that others might be more empathetic to their fellow human than at any time previously. Pour out kindness until it soaks the floor of the planet such that none can take a step without being saturated by the Spirit's righteousness.

Pour my brother. Pour it all out today. Pour out the love you have everywhere you go whenever you are in the company of another. Do not leave anything to chance; make the love you feel for others crystal clear today. Love as though tomorrow offers no guarantees because it doesn't'.

Today, the best of me will spill out wherever I go, and that which is helpful in me, I will offer for the benefit of all others. I am the hose that the Universe supplies eternally. For as long as the Source declares that I must pour, I shall spill out the best of me. For as long as the Spirit fills me with something worth transferring, I will do so continuously.

I will not pour out what is mine personally because anything that is mine is not worth the pour. What is inside me absent from the Creator's mixture of grace and mercy is inferior, insufficient, perhaps even corrupt.

Yet when the Creator disinfects me, only then is what inside me worth pouring out onto others. Only when the Creator sanitizes me am I capable of helping, serving, and making sure others know that their life matters. So, then it is settled, only that which the Creator gives shall I pour and share.

Thank you, Great Spirit, for pouring Your essence in me daily so that I may pour it out onto others. Thank you, Universe, for the opportunity to live this life just as I always imagined. Thank you, Everlasting One, for making me a vessel who shall pour the best of you out of me into the least of these all the days of my life.

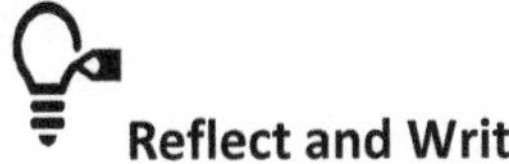

Reflect and Write:

You have spent the last 38 weeks reflecting and writing your way to your best life and the best version of yourself. Now it is time to pour into others.

Because you are on this journey, I suspect you already give of yourself. Yet this week, let's focus our intentions on pouring in a way that will inspire someone else to want to join you on the journey to your best life to the best version of yourself.

Take a moment and think of someone you think could benefit from joining the journey you are on. Write about why you are selecting this person for the journey.

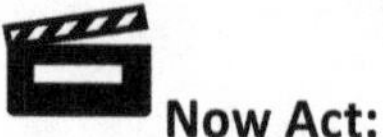

Now Act:

Now choose one of your journal entries from this year. Make a copy of that entry. Write that person who you want to experience this journey and explain to them why you journal forward. Make sure the letter clearly explains why you are sharing your journal entry with them.

After you deliver the letter, watch what occurs as you pour out what is good/great about you through this forward journaling process into them.

Week 40

Keep Going

Good day, Journal,

Keep going! Keep going! I know how you feel. I know darkness and clouds abound right now, but you still must keep going.

Today is no different than any other day. Every day the Universe commands you to keep going. Good times or bad times, you must keep going. High or low moments, you must keep going—no matter who, what, when, where, why, or how, you must keep going.

I mean, after all, what else is there to live for than to keep going. If you stop moving, you die. While you might not die literally, you will die figuratively: emotionally, mentally, and spiritually. If you do not move, you die. Rigor mortis occurs in the mind and spirit just as it does in the body.

If you stop, you cannot grow. So, keep going. Because death's eventuality is inevitable, it's indisputable. If you are not moving, you will soon meet your physical fate if you are not going forward. When your heart and mind stop, your death is certified, the coroner says you are no more; to your family and loved ones, you become only a memory.

I will keep going today because I am nowhere and in no way ready to cease existing. I love my life and all that it is, good and bad times alike. Although if you are listening to me, Universe, I prefer good times a whole lot more. At present, I could use a heaping helping dose of good news and blessed times if it's not asking too much.

Nevertheless, I will keep moving today as the great Dr. King encouraged the nation to do. "If you can't fly, then run, if you can't run, then walk, if you can't walk, then crawl, but whatever you do, you have to keep moving forward."[x]

Yes, sir, Dr. King, I will give all means of moving a try. I will fly when I can, I will run when I cannot fly, I will walk when I am unable to run, and I'll crawl if it's my only option for movement. With cast-iron certainty, you can trust that I will keep moving forward all the days of my life.

Thanks, Dr. King, for the prompt to stay encouraged. Thank you for detailing a process not to get down and out about all the things around us that are out of our control. Thank you for modeling what it looks like to keep the faith when becoming a motionless decaying pessimist would have been so much simpler and easier to do.

It is clear to me that you knew something about moving forward about finding the strength to keep going that most of us still do not understand nor appreciate. Why else would you have bothered when your life could have been so much more straightforward? Why not just move on with your life gracefully, staying in your lane, and merely be a husband and father?

And so, yes, Creator, I hear your voice amplified from the heavens. You did not design me to sit still to be content either. You built me for movement for going places others believe impossible for me to go. Your call on my life is 5G clear; I will keep going until all are helped, served, and made to know that their life matters.

Indeed, to do anything not yet accomplished or that others believe impossible, we must keep going. Keep going and going and going. Keep on moving, don't stop. These are the words of the day.

Yes, I know all the cliches and the accompanying song lyrics to keep going – for moving forward. I know all the cliches and song lyrics because you, dear Creator, place those words and sounds in the deepest recesses of my heart and mind. You position them inside me so that when I feel like quitting, stopping, and giving up, I have a reminder that resigning is not an option for me. I envision the lyrics and hear the music conveying that stopping is unacceptable and that giving up, well, is just blasphemy.

Today, I will keep going, and I will keep moving. I will fly, run, walk, and crawl. I will do whatever it takes to keep moving forward. I will do what I must to fend off rigor mortis. Not just rigor mortis of my body but also the underlying source of rigor mortis that begins in our mind and spirit.

Journey Forward:

Today, I will feed my mind and spirit by living to my full potential by taking in only those things that give my life tremendous meaning. I will read and write words that give others vivacity. I will follow the lead of the Divine spirit by giving and sharing with others. I will express my gratitude for the Universe, which provides and shares with us so kindly and generously.

Today, I will care for my body in the same way that I care for my mind and spirit. I will only consume things that give me the ability to remain 178 pounds of twisted steel with young Denzel sex appeal.

All-day today, I will keep going; I will keep moving. I will fly, run, walk, and crawl to live life as I always imagined. I will fly, run, walk, and crawl to be the best version of myself possible.

Reflect and Write:

If you started this journey of journaling forward at the beginning of the year and have kept pace with the weekly readings, it is now the 10th month of the year. You have made it to October and are hopefully ten months closer to your best life.

Having reached the last quarter of the year, we invite you to take a moment to reflect on how you have grown along this journey. Take a moment and make a list of the ways your life is better today than when you began this journey of journaling forward.

Twelve weeks remain in this year and this journal. This week Nate reminds us that "If you stop, you cannot grow." Thus, for everyone on this journey to live their best lives, we must keep going.

What will you do over the next 12 weeks that you have been putting off? What do you need to change, adjust, and shift to become at the end of the journal whom you promised yourself you would be when you started journaling forward? Write the requisite changes, adjustments, and modifications here.

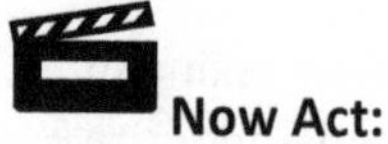

Now Act:

Using Nate's template from the journal, fill in the blank below to get you towards those goals. If you need suggestions on filling in the blanks, look back at Nate's words for ideas.

Today, I will _________________ and ____________________ by living to my full potential by taking in only those things that give my life tremendous meaning.
Today, I will _________________and _________________.
Today, I will care for my ___________________in the same way that I care for my ___________________.

Now post these commitments on your bathroom mirror, refrigerator, car dashboard, anywhere and everywhere to help you keep going this week.

Week 41

Be Accountable

Good day, Journal,

Sure, we have time for one more question. Hell, for as long as we were on lockdown due to COVID-19, feel free to ask all the questions you like. I will only pretend it is 2020 and 2021 again. And thus, say to you, "I got nowhere else to go."

What is the one thing I would advise young people to do to live their best life? That is a genuinely great question.

I can only give them one piece of advice. Let me see. I suppose the one thing I would tell anyone to do is be accountable. To live one's best life, we must make no excuses or allow any room for exceptions.

Yes, I would admonish them about accountability. I am sure you heard me say earlier that I do not like people. But upon further reflection, I suspect I should have instead said, "I truly dislike people. I cannot stand folks who are unaccountable, selfish, and lack self-awareness."

Now that you asked, I further realize that people who are not accountable make me queasy. They make me sick to my stomach. Yes, it is those unaccountable people whom I genuinely dislike.

Folks who say they want a great life but do little or nothing to make it happen. People who would rather blame another for their situation. Persons who prefer not to look themselves in the mirror to assess their actions to find out how they might do better moving forward. Individuals who love to heap the burden of carrying them onto others' shoulders rather than carrying their damn selves. Yep, that's the one thing, accountability.

And the reason I am such a stickler for personal accountability is I was once unaccountable for living the life I always imagined. Yeah, I had a great mantra, "I am healthy, wealthy, and wise. I owe no damn body, period". Yet, I took few if any steps to be who I professed to be in my mantra.

While making this profound affirmation daily, I hypocritically lived. Insecurely, I existed in my disingenuous mantra alleged body. I was overweight. I was out of breath. And the way I was living, I would certainly be out of time soon. I did not act as though the Creator's Temple meant much to me. I was not accountable for my best health.

Health and fitness are the first elements of accountability because I passionately believe that you feel good when you look good. Then when you feel good, you give your all to your life. The better I have looked over the years, the better I felt about myself from head to toe, including mind, body, and spirit.

And this is no bull shit; I have accomplished a whole lot more. I've played the starring role in my life better than ever. I've performed like a star.

But first, I had to get really honest with myself. I had to hold myself, me, and I ultimately accountable. All of me had to participate in the coming to Jesus' meeting, where I first learned that 'Naked Don't Lie, People Do' and 'Fat Meat Is Greasy, But It Ain't Friendly.'

During those coming to Jesus' meetings, I discovered I would need to look in the mirror daily. I would be required to stand on the scale multiple times a day. I would be responsible for counting everything that went inside the Spirit's Spectacular Temple if I ever expected the Temple to look spectacular on the outside.

Finally, when I was ready to be accountable, I got healthy. I mustered the willpower to stop being jealous of the beautiful people in the gym. I got sick and tired of making ridiculous excuses about why I did not have the time or skill set to be at my best. Consequently, I lost forty pounds in six months and prepared for my first bodybuilding contest.

In retrospect, it is no surprise that everything about me changed at that moment. When I proved to myself that I could be one of the beautiful people at the gym, I had evidence that I could be whatever I wanted. I could be who I wanted to be whenever I wanted to be it. Like the fit people in the gym whom I once admired, but now I was amongst those others admired, I knew with certainty that all aspects of my life could be beautiful too.

If I wanted to write, I could write. If I wanted to speak publicly and be compensated for it immensely, I could speak publicly and get paid in full. If I wanted to design planned green communities to change the historically marginalized lives, I could do that very thing.

By holding myself accountable for one thing, my health, I found the catalyst for changing everything else. When I say now that I am in excellent health, maintain abundant wealth, and possess timeless wisdom, it is not just forward-thinking gobbledygook. I do not merely imagine what my best life could be.

Today, I am 178 pounds of twisted steel with young Denzel chocolate sex appeal. I do not owe anybody for real. Money is neither an obstacle nor an excuse for me not to do anything I want whenever I want. Because you all deem me a person in possession of timeless wisdom, I'm allowed to stand in front of this crowd of thousands.

Yes, if you are going to do anything today, become accountable to yourself. Take responsibility for your best life. Do not pass the buck, do not pass go, do not do a damn thing until you first look yourself in the mirror and you do so naked both literally and figuratively.

Ask yourself: Self am I at my best? Self, is this the best I can be? Self, am I living up to my God-given unlimited potential? Self, is this Temple fit for royalty?

If you cannot answer yes to all questions emphatically, you are bullshitting. You are a bullshitter who is wasting preciously gifted undeserved time. You are a bullshitter saying to the Universe you are not only unworthy of, but you don't want any more time.

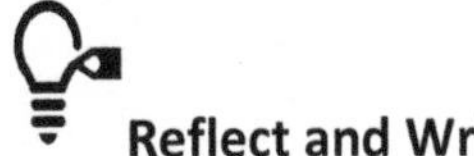

Reflect and Write:

"By holding myself accountable for one thing, my health, I found the catalyst for changing everything else." Take a moment and ask (and answer) yourself this one question, “Am I holding myself accountable for my health?” Write your response.

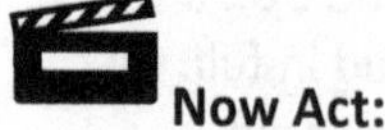
Now Act:

Right now, get naked. Look at yourself in front of a mirror. Answer the following questions: “Self, am I at my best? Self, is this the best I can be? Self, am I living up to my God-given unlimited potential? Self, is this Temple fit for royalty?”

If you cannot answer yes to every question, it’s time for you to set some serious goals related to your health and physical wellness.

With the eleven remaining weeks in this year, take some time to set three SMART goals. These goals will be Specific, Measurable, Attainable, Relevant, and Time-Based.

The time remaining to realize your goals is precisely 11 weeks. Now you just need to execute a strategy that makes you accountable. Try sharing the plans for the final 11 weeks of the year with an accountability partner. Whatever your goals, get to work now.

Week 42

Broken & Better.

Good Day, Journal,

Ernest Hemingway said, "The world breaks everyone, and afterward, some are strong at the broken place." My life is evidence of the integrity of Mr. Hemingway's words.

Boy, oh boy, has the World broken me. The World has broken me too many times to mention. This cold, cruel World like the Hulk has smashed me into millions of pieces.

Still, every time the World's broken me as Legos pulled apart, I realize I can lay around looking a mess. I can continue being a pile of nothing. Or I can see my potential and imagine my best life in the heap of brokenness. Thus far, by the grace of God, I have continued to accept the Universe's gift to begin imagining what is possible for me. I've done so rather than believing being broken is the end of my story.

Each time that the World breaks me, I have gotten up off the ground a mess, no doubt—a complete disaster without question, but I was the total calamity that stood up. I have arisen one more time than the World broke me. I've done so that I might focus my time, attention, and energy squarely on strategizing how to be who I envision.

Like Mr. Hemingway said, "the world breaks everyone." The only difference between legends and the forgotten is that the legendary develop and carry out a plan for their best life. The icons do so in exacting detail. After being broken by the World in an illustrious fashion, those we revere as the exceptional are only so because they chose to adapt themselves to write their story as if right out of Greek mythology.

Like 'The Phoenix' rising, those of us who are broken but refuse to stay broken find a way to fortify ourselves in the broken places so that we are stronger evermore. But to become stronger in the damaged areas, you must admit your weakness. You must not play around or pretend you are healthy when you are weak.

Admission is always the first step to any form of recovery. Admission is the entry fee for becoming more formidable in our broken places.

Before I started to write daily, I was a weak writer. Every teacher and professor said as much. There was never a paper returned to me not marked in red. A 'C' would be a grade to celebrate. 'C' did not mean average to me. A 'C' meant I could celebrate passing.

I was weak. The World had left me broken educationally. But in that pile of 'C' papers with red marks everywhere, with enough red to stop traffic on a busy highway, was a way forward. In my brokenness was a way to become the writer, speaker, Public Intellectual that I would one day hope to be.

In that pile of low grades emphasized by red marks, in that stack of Cs, was a way for me to see my way out. Compiled in mediocrity was a way to see what was possible for me if I committed myself to my desired craft. Sure, I could win awards for writing. Without a doubt, the World could know me as a gifted writer and cunning linguist, but I needed to strengthen my weak writing and speaking aspects. I needed to be authentic with myself about my brokenness.

Today, I am an award-winning author and world-renown speaker. I do not have to tell you about all the awards. You see them on the wall and mantlepiece daily. You know about the calls and requests I receive pleading with me to name my price to come to speak and the publishers all begging to find out what I am writing next.

But it was not that long ago when I exemplified the words of Mr. Hemingway, a man broken by the World. And suppose I am not careful when the World breaks me again, which it surely will because it is what the World does. Shattering people is part and parcel of what the Source created the World to do. In that case, I might stay broken if I did not know better.

Fortunately, I know that being broken is standard. Being broken is an element of the human condition. All humans get harmed; there are no exceptions. All of us get damaged by the World. All of us will be broken time and again.

Journey Forward:

However, when we lay like a pile of brokenness, we must ask ourselves, can I see what is possible? In our sad, pathetic state, like Legos broken into individual bricks, our query should be, do I only see a mess?

When Naeem was a child, he would leave his Legos everywhere. On occasion, he would break whatever he created apart. There would be a pile of seeming nothingness sprawled across the room. Later, as in only a short time, he would return to that pile of brokenness to construct something unique.

Out of nothingness, out of brokenness was a creation we all celebrated. And that is the way I approach life.

Seeing the World as a child sees Legos, I remember what is possible when you put in the work to be your best rather than choosing to see only a pile of brokenness. Envisioning a thing that will make everyone you care about proud rather than perceiving yourself as a pile of brokenness is how you get more robust in the broken places. Visualizing better days ahead is how to fortify yourself after you get broken to live your best life.

Today, I will help, serve, and make sure those broken like me know that being busted up is part of the human condition. Today, I will make sure those broken like me have a process to see how to get up. Today, I will help others broken like me create a strategy for living their life just as they always imagined. Today, I serve as a fortifier for the broken like me to never break in the same way or same place again.

Reflect and Write:

What about Nate's journal resonated with you today? How does being broken relate to where you are on your journey forward, your journey towards being the best version of yourself?

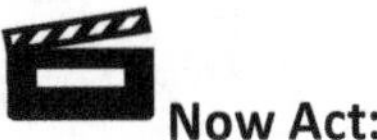

Now Act:

It is time to stop believing being broken is the end of your story. Like the rising 'Phoenix,' those of us who are shattered but refuse to stay broken find a way to fortify ourselves in the broken places so that we are stronger evermore.

Give some thought to what it means to be broken. Do one thing before you go to bed tonight to fortify an area of brokenness in your life.

Week 43

Gangster Tendencies

Good Day, Journal,

Occasionally, the old G.I. comes out. Yep, I am from Gary, Indiana, Gangster Island to those who know G.I. as their hometown. Look, whoever said, "you can leave the island, but the gangster never leaves you," was stone-cold correct. I am G.I. for life, and you better trust and believe that.

Being from G.I. and G.I., being inside me eternally means now, and then I must blast some music with a hardcore bassline. I am serious. It is a necessity.

A solid, predictable root note that gives me pause about how arduous this journey has been. Trust and belief, this journey to be who I always imagined being has not been simple. My life ain't' been no parts easy.

Stacked against me was the deck from the start. There were no silver spoons for me. I might as well keep it one hundred. Sometimes I did not even have a plastic spoon.

You learn a lot from not having proper silverware or plastic utensils. You discover that when you are serious about your life, when a person wants to eat for real, not only will they kill what they eat, but they will eat with their hands.

Listen up, when you are hungry like I am, exceedingly hungry, flat out starving for greatness, whatever gets put before you, you will eat. You will eat it like a gutter rat. Tell'em momma beggars can't be choosers.

That is what it took for me to be a world-famous author and internationally honored Public Intellectual. At times I had to let the G.I. upbringing propel my spirit when the odds were against me when all the walls were closing in on me, urging me to quit. When folks, all those doubters and haters, tried to convince me that this life was not for me that my dreams were absurd, I just took a second to recall my humble G.I. upbringing.

Each time someone tried to convince me to quit, it was as if I invited Big Sean and Chris Brown to perform 'My Last.'[xi] 'My Last' is now one of the songs in my life soundtrack.

(Obnoxiously loud singing, music blasting from my earbuds and oblivious to anyone else while dancing in the sand as I take my morning walk along the beach):

> ♪ Hands up in the air
> I just want the; I just want the baddest b-h in the world.
> Right here on my lap
> And I'ma hit this drink up like it's my last
> I'ma hit this night up like it's my last
> I'ma I'ma, hmm, hmm, like it's my last
> (Boi)
> Swear I'ma, swear I'ma do it like
> Like I never had it at
> All, all, all, all, all, all, all, all
> Like I, like I, like I never had it at
> All, all, all, all, all, all, all, all
> (Boi)
> Like I, like I, like I never had it at
> Boi, boi, hey, okay♪

I cannot begin to count the number of times I gave the critics the middle finger figuratively, most times in my mind but on occasion literally. Quit, I would think mostly to myself because if I said everything that came to my mind, well, let me just say that it might not have been suitable for anyone!

Anyway, what reason would I have to quit? What did I have to lose? I would ask myself each day. I came from nothing. I know better than most what it means to have nothing.

I am not afraid of not having anything. I will never be scared of not having anything. At the end of life, we are all going to a place of nothingness. What I'm afraid of is not trying my best. I'm terrified of not giving my only life my all.

Journey Forward:

I know that unless I do something that matters in the 'here,' I will be nothing in the 'after.' So, I just do what the Creator granted me the time and energy to do daily. Each day, I work my ass off to leave the planet better upon my departure than upon my arrival.

We are keeping it real today, right? In truth, even when it most appeared that I had nothing, I always had something.

I had a fighter's spirit. I had a warrior's tenacity. I had gangster proclivities in my D.N.A. that saturated my existence. I had thuggish inclinations that overrode my programming, no matter how desperately my mother worked to raise me to be a good Christian.

Gangsters are a lot like Christ; they are revolutionary. The best gangsters, like real Christians, care little about having nothing.

Having nothing is the motivation for both groups to have something. Life ever after for Christians, living like this moment is your last for the gangster. And that is the duplicity of the origin story of my G.I. upbringing.

That is why today, I do not live like I am afraid of losing what I have, excellent health, abundant wealth, or timeless wisdom. Today, I live like I have nothing, and tomorrow offers no promises.

Today, I live like I never had 'it,' whatever "it" is at all. Today, I will enjoy the day like it's my last day on this place called earth. Right now, I am going to live, love, and laugh at this moment like it's my last!

> ♪ Man, I just ended up on everybody's guest list.
> I'm just doing better than what everyone projected.
> Knew that I'd be here, so if you asked me how I feel.
> I'ma just tell you; it's everything that I expected, bitch.
>
> Hands up in the air
> (One time for the West Side, West Side let me see them hands)
> Hands up in the air
> (Two times if you love G.O.O.D Music)
> Hands up in the air
> (And three times for the baddest chick in the world)

(Who got her hands up in the air)
Hands up in the air

Now I'ma hit this drink up like it's my last
I'ma, I'ma hit this night up like it's my last
I'ma I'ma, hmm, hmm, like it's my last
Swear I'ma, swear I'ma do it like
Like I never had it at
All, all, all, all, all, all, all
Like I, like I, like I never had it at
All, all, all, all, all, all, all
Like I never had it at all. ♪

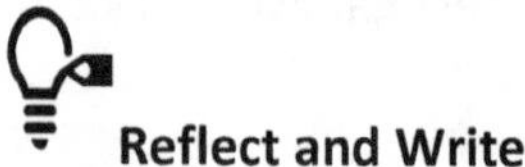

Reflect and Write:

What drives you? What do you care so deeply about that you refuse to quit?

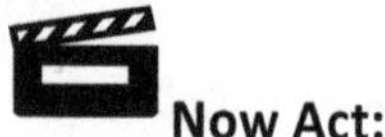

Now Act:

Find a song that you can blast in your earbuds when you consider quitting. Create, if you don't have one already, a "Won't Quit" playlist.

Add this song to the playlist. Be sure to play the songs on the "Won't Quit" list as often as necessary to fuel your "gangster never quit" tendencies.

Week 44

Journal Forward Again!

Good Day, Journal,

How did I get through the Pandemic? I wrote. I scribed a new entry in my journal each day. I wrote whatever came to my mind. Sometimes it was a song, a quote, a feeling, or an emotional connection for which I longed but was unavailable. Notwithstanding, one thing was for sure, I wrote every day.

However, I did not write as most do when writing in their journal. I did not waste time or energy writing about someone who made me angry. Nor did I write about an aspect of society that perturbed me the previous day. Doing either thing would have been a total waste of the preciously gifted time the Universe afforded me.

Because in 2020, there were only a few people I could stand, and there was plenty of stuff that made me angry. If I wanted to write about the tragic past and grim present, I could have quickly done so with little effort. Suppose I wanted to pen words about all the assholes and jerks crossing my path in 2020. In that case, I could have done so with greater simplicity than pushing the Staples "that was easy" button.

But if I started writing down my complaints, when and where would I stop. To what end and to what length would my grievances about people go.

2020 gave us the Pandemic and the irreverent American "know-how" or, more aptly put, American "Don't Know Shit" disease. “Don't Know Shit” disease is the condition of unspeakable stupidity. A disorder that prevented the masses from conceptualizing the importance of wearing a mask to reduce the spread of COVID-19.

Years later, the irony is still not lost on me. We pretentious people, a nation of mask wearers, afraid to let anyone know who we indeed are because we do not know ourselves, objected to wearing a literal mask within stitched the potential to save our and others' lives. A nation of dupes masking their disrespect of humanity behind fake ass arguments of independence while perfectly happy to wear figurative masks and watch their fellow citizens get sick in mass and die alone.

2020 gave us economic collapse that "the haves" celebrated as market growth while the least of these, "the have nots," perished as the bottom of what remained of the so-called American dream fell out. Homelessness and unemployment figures also expanded right in proportion to the ballooning wealth of the elite.

Did I mention the social unrest? American citizens' lascivious behavior included law enforcement called on average Americans bird watching in a public park, folks shot by peace officers while sleeping in their apartment, people assassinated while jogging through the neighborhood, persons walking gleefully out of their garage gun downed by police officers, and regrettably so much more.

Oh, yes! 2020 gave us the Presidential Election and all that goes with a Presidential Election ordinarily. And the 2020 election, just like everything else about 2020, was anything but typical. There was truly little about the Election for a new Commander in Chief that was either conventional or presidential.

Life usually is depressing enough for me without a Pandemic, especially during the winter months. Thus, keeping a traditional journal during the winter months in Indiana combined with COVID-19 could have been enough to believe there was nothing for which to be hopeful. So, as I said, I wrote about everything but not that which was occurring in real-time.

Dark days both literally and figuratively. Damp and cold days repeatedly. An external and internal climate ripe for one suffering from SAD (Seasonal Affective Disorder). A debilitating mental and horrifying emotional fusion prepared by America to give one severe thought of not only being somewhere else on the planet but leaving this fucking planet for the great beyond altogether with the quickness.

Thus, as I said, I wrote about things that could improve my disposition. I wrote about my best life, which I do not believe is a coincidence, is the exact life I live today. I do trust we are what we think. And in 2020, I changed the way that I thought so that I might not merely change the way I lived but that I might also like the 'Five Heartbeats'[xii] feel like going on.'

I changed what I believed was occurring so that I might live as I always imagined. I gave my time and energy to imagining my best life so that I might soon live my best life. I reflected intently and religiously on being the best version of myself so that I might best help, serve, and make sure others know that their life matters.

Now that 2020 is in the rearview mirror, appearing as an object closer than it truly is, I still write in my journal. I always journal forward. I continue reflecting on life as I imagine it as I desire it to be, not as it is. I do so, especially if what I am experiencing in the flesh does not match what I dream of in my heart and mind.

'I Journaled My Way Forward Through 2020.' I made it through one of the worst periods in the world's history by making up a righteous, personally beneficial history in my mind. I journaled forward this morning, and should the Creator grant me the opportunity, I will journal forward tomorrow as well.

I journal forward because I know that seeing my best life in my minds' eye and then writing that life down is the first step to living the life I always imagined. The journaling forward is my life blueprint, a blueprint from the Universe to construct my best life right here and right now. It is when I journal forward that my heart pulsates, and I feel like going on.

Reflect and Write:

Take a moment and reflect on how the events of 2020 affected you. Now that 2020 is behind you, in hindsight, what would you do differently?

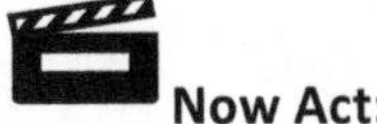

Now Act:

What's your plan for when things are hard? How will you react differently than in 2020? Consider taking all the ways you wished you were different in 2020 and apply them to your life now.

Write yourself a letter to be opened by you six months from today. Report in the letter how you responded to the most recent adversity in your life.

Week 45

Lessons Learned

Good Day, Journal,

Ah, Hawaii! Hawaii is the kind of word that simultaneously oozes out of your mouth and soothes your soul. Not a lot of words do that for me. Only the rarest words give my tongue and lips joy as they pass through my mouth while simultaneously warming my heart and soul.

But Hawaii does that for me. Hawaii gets me every time. Hawaii gives it to me all the time.

I do not know what it is about being here precisely. It could be all the leis (pronounced lays) I am offered.

No, get your head out of the gutter. I am talking about the wreath of flowers. I'm referencing the floral bouquet strung together and placed around your neck—the expression of humanity gifted to a visitor upon arriving or leaving. A symbolic necklace of affection from the native people is the leis.

Perhaps it is the music featuring string instruments like ukuleles. I am just not sure I can put my finger on it, but whatever it is, I completely love it here.

There was a time when I was not sure I would ever get here. I purchased a trip in early February 2020 to come here for the first time. And wouldn't you know it, COVID-19 struck and derailed those plans. Eight days and seven nights in a three-bedroom ocean suite canceled just like that. Thanks, Pandemic. Thanks for nothing, 2020.

Talk about a real bummer. Yet, using the word 'bummer' is mainly how the majority describe 2020. As we look back on 2020, though maybe with rose-colored glasses, I think that year taught us a lot about who we are and what we want out of this thing called life.

I cannot speak for everyone else, but in 2020 I learned more about myself than I ever knew previously. Life slowed down, allowing me an unprecedented opportunity to do some much-needed self-examination. Something about a global pandemic, the likes of which the world had not seen in a century, changes the way people look at life and the world.

It is hard to take tomorrow for granted when so many people are suffering and dying each day. It is nearly impossible to pretend you are genuinely alive, living the life you always imagined when you are not sure you or those you love and adore will be around much longer. Believing you are the best version of yourself is an absolute absurdity when nothing about the world is even close to its best.

If there is any singular positive universal thing to take away from 2020, I suppose it was the realization that we all need to live in the moment. 2020 taught us that it was past time to start loving and laughing so much more purposely, intensely, and deeply. It was time to love our neighbor as ourselves for real. The time was upon us to finally extend the best of humanity to the least of these.

Before 2020, I think families and friends took each other for granted. I'm relatively confident we all took the gift of the Universe's present for granted. Sadly, most of us have returned to our old unappreciative, heartless, foolishly living as if tomorrow offers promises selves.

But in 2020, some of us learned, or at least I did, to use the new day to be a better version of myself than yesterday's edition. I also discovered which family members and friends were the real keepers and which ones I could and must exclude from my life.

Oh yes, 2020, the year that canceled my first planned trip to Hawaii, laid the groundwork for me to spend three or more months each year right here in Hawaii. As I said, everything about 2020 was not terrible.

These days I do not get as many leis as I did when I first started coming here. Again, get your head out of the gutter. I get fewer bouquets because most of the native people know me. I am less like a guest and instead 'play cousin' if you will, kind of an honorary member of the extended indigenous Hawaiian family.

Journey Forward:

I cannot tell you how much I adore the people here. Their hospitality reminds me of the good old Southern charm without the fear of folks wearing white bedsheets and planting flaming crosses at night. And when they offer to put something around my neck, it's a 'lei,' not a noose.

Oh yes, Hawaii! Fresh vegetation is everywhere. Sunshine in epic proportion. Refreshing, beautiful waterfalls all over the place. Hawaii is indeed a tropical paradise.

Ain't that something, paradise, as in the phrase I often used to express how I felt during 2020. When asked how I was or how things were going, my usual response was "just another day in paradise." Back then, I was not even close to paradise's physical or geographic vicinity. Still, I found a way to be in this heavenly place in my mind.

I guess it is true if you tell yourself something long and often enough, you start to believe it. I surmise that it is also true that it becomes your reality if you think something dreamt of as real long enough. And now here I am, in this little place of the world that I call paradise.

Paradise where people treat me like I matter. Paradise where the sun, sand, palm trees, and ocean are ubiquitous. Paradise where each day, when asked how I'm doing, I can honestly state, "Today is just another day in paradise!"

Reflect and Write:

What are the things you promised to do differently when the pandemic was over? How are you doing at keeping your promises? Be specific. Give yourself a grade on each completed pledge.

Now Act:

Choose one area that you graded yourself a C or less. Now devise a plan on how to keep and honor your promises.

Share your promises with your accountability person. Ask them to check on your progress weekly until the end of the year.

Week 46

A Way to Say Thank You

Good Day, Journal,

Hello Great Spirit! I see you! I know what you have going on today.

I feel your presence peeking through the clouds. I have that feeling today you will cascade your Supreme essence over me all day long. So, let me say it while it is fresh on my mind. Thank you! Thank you so very, very much.

Trust and believe that I will be saying thank you again and again throughout the day. I know without you, there is no me. I realize that I am but a vessel. A container lacking your presence would be empty. Without your grace and mercy beneficently pouring the best of you inside me, my cup would at best runneth over with mediocrity.

To be sure, I know full well that nothing you do is average. Neither is anything that comes from you less than great.

What is average, then? Where does mediocre originate? Lackluster then is our failed interpretation and misuse of your gifts.

The gifts of time, free will, aspiration, independent thinking, and more are not average gifts. The presents you supply in abundance are phenomenal. You give so lavishly, and for whatever reason, we perform and utilize your unjust rewards and undeserved offerings so poorly. Regrettably, we make incredible miracles look like ordinary trash.

But today, at least for one day, I will not misuse your gifts. I cannot promise what I will do tomorrow as you have not promised me another day. However, today, I can tell you that I will not waste the precious time you have so generously shared.

I will begin the day taking care of your magnificent Temple. A body so few cherish appropriately, but one I recognize is on par with any of the best gifts you endow.

I will eat right today, staying at or below my 1,500 designated calories. I will consume my gallon of water. I will have my required 150 or so grams of protein as prescribed for my best health. My high-intensity interval training and cardio will last no less than 60 minutes.

Of course, I will begin my day, as I do daily, standing naked on the scale. Looking at the digital reading, glancing at myself in the mirror, I'm assured neither does the scale or au naturel lie.

People lie, but today, I will be honest as the scale. I dare not lie to myself. I bare myself to the naked truth: I am supposed to remain 178 pounds of twisted steel with young Denzel chocolate sex appeal.

On this day, I will put the gift of wisdom to excellent use. I will exercise great judgment, refusing to buy anything that is not an absolute necessity. I will not spend in excess or fool myself into thinking I deserve to treat myself to something expensive or inexpensive, for that matter.

I will save more than I spend even though tomorrow offers no promises. For I know the Wise One expects us to do what is best to prepare adroitly should tomorrow come. Therefore, if the Universe grants me a tomorrow like a squirrel, I will have some nuts stashed away just in case. Like the person with extra roof tiles to patch up a hole, I will save some tile for a rainy day. A rainy day that life has shown me time and again is inevitable.

Thank you, Universe! Thank you for this day. I do not care how many more times I say thank you; it will not be enough. It matters not how redundant those two words may seem; I will not cease speaking them.

Thank you for waking me this morning, allowing me to be in what I believe is in my right mind. Thank you for allowing my heart and mind to operate at peak efficiency. Thank you for what others take so for granted, the sunlight beaming off my face and skin. Thank you for the sand beneath my feet and each wonderful golden-brown grain stuck between my toes.

Journey Forward:

If you allow me, I would like to give an extra special thank you. Thank you for keeping me on task. Thank you for reminding me to live every moment in the present while meeting the expectation never to lose sight that the present moment does not belong to me singularly. In each present moment, I am part of the great universal reciprocal circle of life.

Today, I will carry out the incompletable mission of helping, serving, and making sure others know that their life matters. For this, I know! No matter how many people I helped, served, and made sure they knew that their life counted yesterday or today, tomorrow there will be millions in need of reassurance that, like me, they know their lives have a purpose.

By no means does their purpose require them to do or become what I have become a renowned Public Intellectual, international philanthropist, and Humanity Propulsion Engineer. Instead, the universal life purpose is finding our unique way to leave the planet better upon our departure than on our arrival.

Thank you for allowing me to be a helper, a servant, and a confidant to others, most notably the least of these! Thank you for gifting me the life I have always imagined living! Thank you for prepping me daily to be the best version of myself possible! Thank you! Thank you! Thank you!

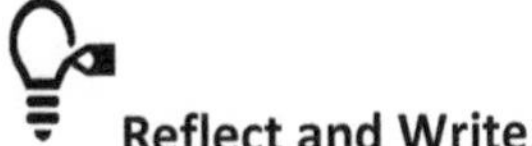

Reflect and Write:

Read back through Nate's plans for showing gratitude and appreciation for the gifts given to him today. Do you have a similar to-do or action list?

What might you complete on your list today? What else should you add to your list?

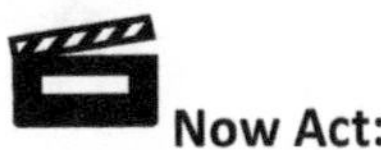

Now Act:

Using Nate's list as a guide, write your list that will show your gratitude for the gift of life. Stay focused only on what you will do today.

Revisit the list to see how you did at the day's end. Adjust your list for tomorrow, accordingly tomorrow.

Week 47

Die Trying

Good day, Journal,

Phew! What a day! What a life! Now that the Pandemic is behind us, the possibilities of living our best life again are upon us all.

Truthfully, the possibility of living our best life never left. The only thing disappearing during the Pandemic was our willingness to believe that the best is not only yet to come, but the best is always here.

The Universe gives us the most profound opportunity to live an extraordinary life every single solitary day. Pandemic or nothing but clear mask-free skies, we have the choice every day in every way to live life just as we always imagined. No matter what is going on outside or around us, life can be extraordinary.

The trick to living your best life to living the life you always imagined, even during the worst of times like a Pandemic, is to believe in doing the impossible. When you believe in doing the impossible, you establish first in your mind that nothing and no one can stop you. With unbreakable mental, emotional, and spiritual conviction, you know that not even the worst Pandemic in a hundred years can stop you from doing the impossible.

During the Pandemic, I realized that I was at a crossroads. I could sink or swim. Sink in the abyss of the Pandemic and all the sickness, death, and sadness about me was one option. Or I could learn to swim across the Divine channel of great possibilities was the other option.

Because the Creator requires me to be honest, I must state that there were days when I quite frankly wanted to give up. There were more than a few days when I tried convincing myself that I did not care if I sank to the bottom of the abyss.

Fortunately, on more days than not, I wanted to swim. I had to swim because swimming was the only thing that would keep me from dying. Swimming was the only thing that would get me across to the other side – the place called joy and happiness.

When you want to succeed as bad as I want to be continuously successful, you learn to "suck it up." "Suck it up," meaning to get your heart, mind, and spirit right and put in work during life's most debilitating moments. "Suck it up," as in placing your head on straight, remembering that your life is more significant than to just you. "Suck it up" and jump in the deep end first.

I have learned two things about jumping in the deep part that are preeminent reasons for my prolific success as a writer and prolonged staying power as a Public Intellectual. First, if you are going to fail, you might as well meet your fate honorably if you are going to die. You might as well die trying to do something audacious.

How embarrassing would it be to fail at swimming while in the shallow end of the pool? How hard would you have to try to sink to drown in the part of the water nearest the shore?

Failing is one thing but not giving your best effort is worse than failing. Choosing the easy way out and still falling flat on your ass is downright unacceptable. Failing because you did not give your maximum effort makes you an abomination to the Creator.

The second thing jumping in the deep end taught me is that once you make it across the pool from the deep end to the shallow end, you can no longer subscribe to the idea that 'impossible' is real. When you do the audacious once and succeed, you have eternal evidence, lifetime proof that the impossible is nothing. From that day forward, subsequently and always, the impossible is meaningless forever!

Impossible means nothing to me now, so I routinely look for the most audacious things to do. For some, I dream what is unimaginable because, in my mind, I know the impossible does not exist.

All thoughts and ideas are possible for the person who is not afraid to leap into the deep end of the pool. Everything is achievable for the one who does the unimaginable merely once.

Journey Forward:

So, this Thanksgiving, several 'Thanksgiving Days' removed from the horrific 2020 Thanksgiving, I express my everlasting appreciation to the Creator for convincing me that it is not only okay, but it is best if I leap into the deep end of the pool. Today, I happily throw caution where it best belongs to the wind.

Today, I live with unbridled passion and joy because the Universe did not design either love or pleasure with restrictor plates. Like driving a Formula One race car, passion and joy are best when steered unrestrained by fear, navigated to the winner's circle, and experienced peddle entirely flat on the metal.

Passion, joy, and dreaming are gifts from the Universe that magnify that we are alive. And the more unrestrained we allow them to be, the more amplified and vibrant we know we are.

I am alive right now, and I know it because I can feel it way down deep in my soul. Lookout 'deep end,' here I come again!

Nate wrote, "You might as well die trying to do something audacious." Share your thoughts.

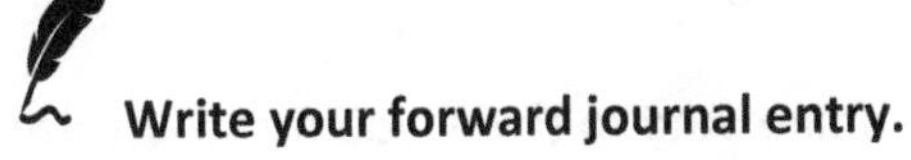

What do you believe the following year's version of you will say a year from now about the audacious things you have accomplished in the past year? Today journal forward about at least one thing you won't die without trying!

Week 48

Be GREAT

Good Day, Journal,

It is time! It is time to get up and get going. Yeah, I know it is still dark outside. I believe this time of day is what is called pitch dark. Pitch dark or not, it is nonetheless time. It is time for you to rise and shine!

Rise and shine, what an interesting phrase. Rise as in you first must get up. It would be best if you rose from slumber.

You must climb even higher when you fall or get knocked down. It is not merely enough to reach your initial intended step. You must show others that you are inevitable. You must go beyond that original expectation. Whatever you do, you must recognize that before you can shine, you must rise.

Shine as in as the kids say, "flossing." Shine, you must do like a new penny. Pennies shining or not shining are not something you see much these days. Nowadays, few of us use anything other than digital currency.

Still, like a newly minted penny, you must shine. And to shine, you first must rise and then do all the things that bring a shine not only to your life but a deep brilliant luster to others. Humanity sparkles best when you help, serve, and make sure others know their life matters when the brilliance of others is permitted to glow and grow.

I realize you could lay around today. You could sleep in past noon. Lollygagging for as long as you want and still see your bank account grow but is that you? Is that what you are about, only dollar-dollar bills y'all?

I got to be honest with you; that person whose day I just described above is someone for whom I am unfamiliar. Do you recall who you said you wanted to become long ago? Have you forgotten the days when you did not have either the pot or the window to discard your piss? Do you remember how you said you want the planet to recognize you after the last grain of sand drips from the top half of your life hourglass?

Let's see if memory serves me correctly. Aren't you the guy who encourages one packed audience after another week after week to live this life as though we are intentionally writing our obituary? Isn't it you who stands before a packed house asking questions of all attendees? Don't you demand that all of us give our total consideration daily to living a life that matches what we'd like said in our eulogy?

This life, as you tell others, is not a dress rehearsal. We must then utilize this life as our one opportunity to say to the world decisively who we are. This thing we know as life, an aliveness that the Universe wants us to experience fully as our best life, can indeed be so.

We must understand that to shine, we need first raise our self-expectations. We must rise daily and do an incredible amount of sometimes exhausting quantities of work.

So, rise. Rise and be great today. Be the expression of remarkable that you tell Naeem about consistently.

Be G.R.E.A.T. Be GOOD to yourself. RESPECT the Universe's wondrous gift of the present. EXEMPLIFY the best of humanity in both word and deed. ASPIRE to live your life just as you always imagined. TREAT others, including friends, family, neighbors, to distant cousins, with double the love and adoration you desire in your life.

Rise and be GREAT today. Only when you rise and make the commitment to be GREAT can you expect to shine. Only after you wake gratefully and choose to put in a GREAT effort today purposely is it even possible for you to shine.

If you need any more incentive to get out of bed despite how dark it remains outside, here's a little word from the Sponsor. A shining star, which is what you are, shines brightest in the dark.

So, get up and get going. Get up and go to work while it remains dark so that you may both manifest your best life and brightly shine so that others may see that the way to be their best self begins while it is dark.

Today, I will rise. I will advance further than planned, even if I fall. No matter how many times I fall or get knocked down, I will spread my wings, soar, and keep moving forward.

Today, I am up, and I am GREAT. Today, I am up, and not only am I better than ever, but I am also Universe blessed GREAT.

Today, I shall shine like no time previously. I will shine as a living example of the Universe's power and intentions. I will be a shining example of one who understands that we only get one shot at life. To hit life's bullseye, we must rise, be GREAT, and shine ubiquitously (helping, serving, and making sure others know that their life matters).

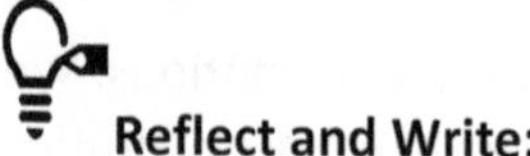

Reflect and Write:

What will you do to be GREAT today? Write it here in detail.

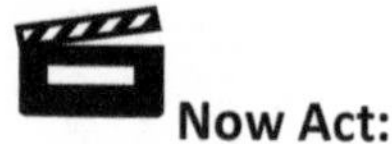

Now Act:

Write the following down in large print. Place it in a location where you can see and recite it throughout the day as a reminder of your commitment to Be GREAT!

> *Be G.R.E.A.T. Be GOOD to yourself. RESPECT the Universe's wondrous gift of the present. EXEMPLIFY the best of humanity in both word and deed. ASPIRE to live your life just as you always imagined. TREAT others with double the love and adoration you desire in your life.*

Invite others to join you in the quest to Be GREAT today to Be GREAT every day!

Week 49

Be Fear Fueled

Good Day, Journal,

Can I let you in on a little secret? Audience participation is my favorite part of public speaking. I thoroughly enjoy this part because you – the audience, fans, and detractors – push me to think differently to give the common social issues a much more profound reflection.

So, you want to know how I became so courageous. Well, what if I told you that I am not courageous at all. More than anything, I am fueled by fear. I know many who believe fear is an acronym. F.E.A.R. as in false evidence appearing real.

Fear, however, for me, is a type of fuel like hydrogen fuel. Fear propels me to do things others, including myself, believed were impossible at one time or another. Like hydrogen fuel, fear is a compound no different than hydrogen and oxygen readily accessible, waiting for proper utilization.

Who do I fear? No human. There is no man or woman that I fear. Who I fear is the broader you? I fear letting you, the inhabitants of the planet, down by not living up to my potential. I fear leaving this planet an adulterated mess because I was not courageous enough to be the best version of myself possible.

Yes, my fear is about something bigger than me – each one of you. It is my solemn hope and dream that you would let fear drive you the same way it moves me. I wish more people would be afraid of not living each day to the maximum. I want the masses to fear not doing all they can to leave the planet better upon our departure than upon our arrival.

Fear even directs my diet and fitness goals. I fear not being 178 pounds of twisted steel with young Denzel chocolate sex appeal. It is fearing not being at my healthiest that drives me to do what is required to feel better about myself to love what I see when I look at myself naked in the mirror. I heard Deion

Sanders say, "If you look good, you feel good. If you feel good, you play good. If you play good, they pay good".

I take care of myself similarly because I know that looking and feeling my best is the only way to make a worthwhile and lasting contribution to society. Taking great care of myself is the only way to win the mental, physical, and spiritual Olympics of life.

I do not want to be a drudge of society. I do not want to be a figurative societal hobo with my hat held out, waiting for another to do what I can and should do for myself. So, I do what is necessary, not because I am courageous but because I fear the alternative.

Fear is not the opposite of courage. For me, fear fuels courage. I so fear letting people down that I have no option but to then do what appears courageous.

You may wonder why I am telling you this. Why is this man spilling the beans about his fear? Well, first, I am attempting to answer the audience member's question authentically. Secondarily, I want you to find the thing you are fearful of, that great regret you would have if you learned you were out of time, and let that thing fuel your progress.

I am sure there are those of you in the audience who are now, as I was not long ago—people looking for a way to be better. Folks, simply hoping to live a life of real significant meaning. People, now searching for a sign that would enable you to live your life just as you always imagined finally. Well, here is the signpost.

Be fearful! Fear wasting the generously gifted time you have right now—fear doing anything less than striving to be the best version of yourself. Fear having to answer to the Creator why, although gifted with so much talent, you left untapped most of it. Fear knowing that you were here on this planet for however many years you've been here, and up until now, if you left, few if anyone would even know you were here in the first place.

Today, please have the courage to want to leave a mark on the planet so that the world will miss you? Be courageous enough to use fear to propel you forward. So that even if you miss the moon, you, like other greats boosted by fear, land exactly where you are supposed to be upon the stars. Fear leaving up to others what the Creator designed you to do – to help, serve, and make sure others know their life matters.

Reflect, Write, and Now Act:

"Fear having to answer to the Creator why, although gifted with so much talent, you left untapped most of it." ~NT Write what these words mean to you.

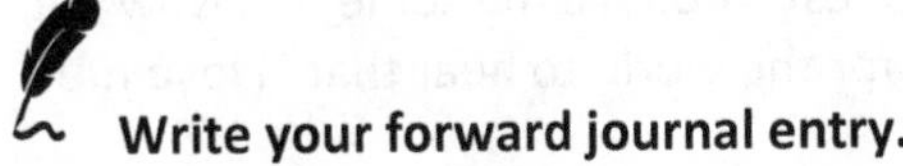

Write your forward journal entry.

At this time next year, what will you have to say about how you used fear to fuel your efforts to live your best life? Journal forward about how fear propelled you forward!

Week 50

Love Me Some Me

Good day Journal,

I love me some me! I am serious. I do. I honestly do love me some me. Now and then, it bears saying repetitively out loud for the world to hear that "I love me some me."

There are times where I must scream it out loud from the top of my lungs now and again as a reminder, primarily to myself, that I love me some me. I cannot overstate the importance of self-love.

Self-love is especially crucial for anyone with designs on loving another. Self-love is undeniably essential for anyone tasked as we all are with helping, serving, and making sure others know that their life matters. In short, self-love intends to be the outward manifestation of loving all humanity.

Notwithstanding the overwhelming degree to which I love myself today, I dare not act as though I always loved myself. I will not put on any pretentious airs on this day or any other. Like so many Americans, I am a product of a society built on only the tiniest minority of people taught that they should and must love themselves openly and authentically.

Even today, I am a citizen victimized continuously by a sometimes-hollow Declaration. This national pronouncement restricts self-love by the least of these. A citizen who does not always enjoy the independence to experience the full rights and privileges of said citizenship, a societal responsibility built on a love of self.

A citizen who, despite this nation's shortcomings, will never stop loving himself. A citizen whose love of self inspires him to hold on to and pursue the self-evident Spiritual truths of life, liberty, and the pursuit of happiness relentlessly. I have come to understand life, freedom, and joy in a fashion none can ever experience absent self-love.

Journey Forward:

I am telling you there was so much about my identity, humanity that I did not love. I also suspect one could surmise that I despised myself. From the top of my head to the soles of my feet, I found extraordinarily little about me worth loving. Once upon a time, there was no love of self at all.

I could not stand my hair because it was kinky, just too damn nappy. At times, even my family would unconsciously refer to my locks maliciously. The result was that I was not too fond of my mane right along with them.

Who could love hair associated with a wooly mammoth? Who would love themselves when a 'Brillo Pad' was their hair's closest comparison? Who could be said to love their hair when they put chemicals in it to change its natural texture to match that of another?

Today, being follicly challenged and increasingly gray, I would give almost anything for a full head of the nappiest and kinkiest hair ever. Not a single chemical would I add to its natural state. I would embrace my hair like never previously because today I love me some me.

I had no love for my lips. Too broad, too big my lips were. My childhood friends would call me "Bubblicious," as in the bubblegum. Regularly hurled at me were derogatory names such as big-lipped, juicy fruit lips, big old African lips, and helium lips.

I did not understand then that my big lips were defining attributes of my glorious ancestral origin. Back in the day, like those family members and friends making fun of me, I did not love myself enough to appreciate my God-given uniqueness.

Today, I love my lips not because they kiss up to others or because "full" lips are now fashionable. I love my lips nowadays because I understand their origin and their connection to my humble and honorable beginnings.

Even the color of my skin, often fraught with horror for some, is no longer something that troubles me. Again, truth is powerful, so I must speak honestly.

There was a short period when I wondered if God, allegorically, cursed me as a mythical descendant of Ham. I pondered if my color was a lifetime penalty for the fictional sin of someone I did not know personally.

Today, I do not believe in such deceitful Biblical nonsense. Nor that the Creator would penalize me for another's action, much less the misdeeds of someone I did not know. Moreover, and perhaps equally important, I do not ascribe to a belief that anyone is inferior or superior to another.

In the Creator's eyes, I know we are all equally unique and similarly unremarkable. I know that we are all equally beautiful and ugly, and nonetheless, we are still loved by the Source comparably. That's why these days, I'm able to declare for any who will listen that “I love me some me.”

Furthermore, I pray that all of us learn to love ourselves equally. Because until we learn to love ourselves entirely and accept who we are uniquely on the outside, there is no way to love anyone, much less ourselves.

Without the love of self, no one can be their best; none of us can live our best life. Deprived of self-love, we can do no more than become the thieves who steal from the world the best possible versions of ourselves.

Self-love is the compensation we owe the Universe for loving us first. Self-love makes the world go round. Self-love is best for all humanity.

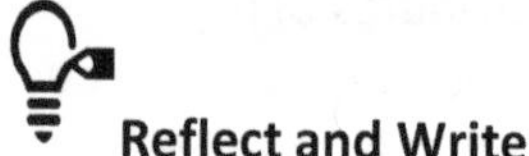

Reflect and Write:

What do you LOVE about yourself? Make a list. What is it about the characteristics/traits you chose that you love? Be both specific and detailed.

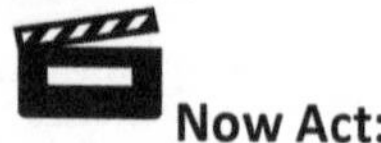

Now Act:

You guessed it! It’s time for you to Journal forward. Include in your entry things the future you will love the most about YOU as you become the best version of yourself. Be specific!

Journey Forward:

Week 51

Get Out of Your Way

Good day Journal,

Yes, of course, you may ask a question. Feel free to ask anything you like. I am, after all, an open book. I find it so much easier to be transparent than to try to figure out what the hell you said or did not say the last time you spoke about the same subject.

"How do you get out of your way to be who you always dreamt of being?" Wow! Now, is that ever a loaded question. Perhaps I should rethink my strategy of being transparent. As usual, it seems I might have bitten off more than I can chew. We are here now, so let us throw caution to the wind.

I suppose there's much advice one could give, but I find the direct route as it is, in most things, the best approach. Straight talk, no chaser is the way I like to speak. So here goes!

If I understand it correctly, your query seems to include a caveat. You are blocking your path, prohibiting your journey, delaying the prospects of arriving at your best life. So, if my assumption is correct regarding the caveat, the most important thing you must do is move out of the way. You must get out of your damn way!

Without delving deeply into the question and its relation to one's life directly, I recommend taking a high-quality long pause. Define specifically and emotively where you want to go. Furthermore, I would implore you to decide who you want to be. Put all bullshit aside, give direct testimony to the Universe regarding where you are currently and who you are right here, right now.

When those two points in one's life spectrum, who you are now and whom you desire to be, are not aligned, you know your life is out of whack. You know you are in your way.

Journey Forward:

This getting genuine part of living is the aspect most people want no part of doing. Folks love to talk about keeping it real. But rarely do we keep it honest about who we are and why we are wherever we are.

We hardly ever keep it one hundred. Even when deliberating something as simple as why are we are not living up to our potential, we remain counterfeit. Pretenders we are when the query is if we are living life just as we always imagined.

Like most things I discuss, my understanding of these issues comes from my own experience. I know this to be an indisputable truth. Most of us are not where we want to be or wish others will remember us as having existed when we are gone because we are stuck in time.

We are stuck in time, as in still living in the past. Stuck, we are in the past of our childhood upbringings. Rooted, like an old tree, are the masses in the history of a previous bad relationship. Like everyone I know, moored to a preceding life event where no one wants to be because the outcome is not what we want.

No matter who the world thinks we are or what we have done to date, we often get in our way. Routinely, we rush to stand in the path of a promising bright future by living in the past. Like a graphic novel character with a tumultuous background narrative, we must learn that our origin story will not change.

However, depending on how we live each day, the way our origin story is perceived can change. There is beauty in an origin story. No matter how bad the start, we can become who we once thought impossible. We can also encourage others to believe in the possibilities of their lives as well.

If you come from an abusive household where a parent mentally, physically, or emotionally abuses you for the bulk of your childhood, that story cannot change. Trust me. I know that story personally. That story is dry and firm as cement.

There is not a damn thing you can do about the past. The past, like a city cement sidewalk, is paved. However, what you control is the future and whether or not you live the present so that your origin story rouses or inhibits your future.

Some of us take the shit from our past and treat it like a bioengineer uses manure. We turn the muck of life into biofuel. We let the bullshit from our history energize us to live the life of our dreams. We take the manure dished out on us repeatedly and turn the excrement into a source of power.

I think you must learn to do this first and foremost. You must stop thinking of your origin as anything more than the beginning of your story. Unless I missed out on 'Storytelling 101', the opening is not the end. Until the lights go out in your eyes until the beat stops in your heart, you are not at the end, and there is still plenty of life to be lived and stories to be written and told.

Today, choose to get out of your way. Join me and commit as we are all called to do daily to get out of our way so that we might live our best life.

Whether the past was good or bad is inconsequential. The fact that we are alive now means gone is yesterday. Thus, today is a day to live in the moment, a moment of striving to get to the destination of our choosing and being the best version of ourselves possible.

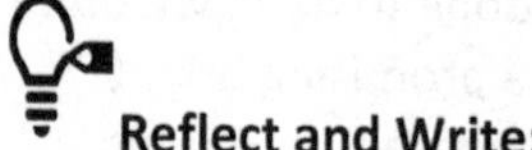

Reflect and Write:

Let's do what Nate suggests precisely. I would recommend taking a high-quality long moment to define specifically and emotively where you want to go and who you want to be. Put all bullshit aside, give direct testimony to the Universe regarding where you are currently and who you are right here, right now."

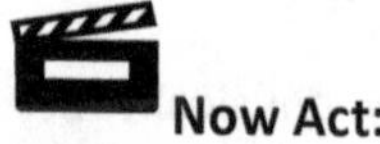

Now Act:

Journal forward, answering the question below the way you would answer from your best life perspective. "How do you get out of your way to be who you always dreamt of being?"

Week 52

Competition

Good day Journal,

Boy, oh boy! You thought the tricky part was climbing, but you now know that the climb is the easiest part. The hard part, the excruciatingly difficult part few people talk about, is staying.

Staying at the top of the peak is far more challenging than climbing the mountain. Not to say climbing to the highest professional elevation is easy. I'm merely stating that staying on top presents an entire set of challenges you could not understand until you are here.

When you are at the bottom of the mountain, it is easy to see how high you must climb when lying low in the valley, are you! The terrain that you must climb is prominent. The obstacles and obstructions are in plain sight.

But what you cannot do from the bottom of the mountain is appreciating what it will be like once you get to the top. It is also not possible to conceive while free climbing life's perilous mountainous journey how challenging the fight it is to stay on top.

For sure, when you get here, it is euphoric. To say one is overjoyed is an understatement. Whatever the words are for being beyond delighted and ecstatic, take those words and multiply them by a thousand.

I am not exaggerating. The experience is indeed all of that! The only thing close to the incredible delight of reaching the mountain top was watching Naeem being born and holding him for the first time.

I remember Naeem's cone head like his birth was yesterday and the regal nature for which he entered the world. For sure, on June 27, 1995, I was ecstatic and euphoric.

There I go using incommensurate words again. Once more, I need better words much more descriptive expressions to accurately describe what I felt.

But that genuinely is kind of what it felt like to get to the mountain top. To look around and see how high you have climbed. To look down to see how far you have come—taking note of all it took to get here.

To notice those people like you once were now looking up to you from the bottom. Taking a moment to view all those following in my path, attempting to complete the same climb.

All of it would be somewhat surreal if you were not a believer in the Universe. Perhaps if you thought the impossible was a reality, surreal might be the appropriate thought and feeling.

Yet, you know the moment is real because you know how hard you worked. You know you gave when you were empty. You know you shared even when you were broke. You know you like the little red engine, singly believed you could, and solo, you kept going.

Still, after the euphoria passes and the overjoy subsides, there is a terrifying reality. You still must work. Your best life continues to demand that you work your ass off. Because if you do not work, you will soon find others treating you like a shipwrecked Gilligan. They will be trying to get you off the Island.

The reservation to the 'Island of Greatness' is an honor for those willing to work every day. The 'Island of Greatness' can be a short respite or a lifetime home. If you arrive and how long you reside there is totally up to you.

In this your only life, you can choose to be a one-hit-wonder or a wonder who repeatedly provides hits to the world. But, again, once you are on top of the mountain, who you are going forward is up to you. Your decisions determine the length and quality of your stay.

So, what does it take to stay on top of the mountain? Who gets to remain on top, looking down and around at the glorious sights and others nipping at your feet trying to replace you? The answer is more straightforward than folks think.

Journey Forward:

The actions and behaviors of others are of no consequence. The accomplishments or achievements of others mean nothing. You are not in competition with anyone but yourself.

You are competing with yourself day after day, hour after hour, and minute after minute. Staying on top requires the same relentless pursuit of excellence that you gave during the climb. To continue living in excellent health, possessing abundant wealth, and sharing timeless wisdom, means you must challenge yourself to a duel—the duel against complacency.

Will the version of you on the top of the mountain win out, or the edition of you who believes what happened yesterday matters not? I place my money and faith in the competitor that the Universe trusts, the dissatisfied, always pissed off at complacency, ravenously hungry, "I have done nothing yet" version.

Now it is up to you to choose who will you be today? Whom will you be for the 86,400 seconds endowed to you by the Source? The guy who made it to the top and became complacent or the guy who knows there remains a lifetime of climbing still to do?

Reflect and Write:

The actions and behaviors of others are of no consequence. The accomplishments or achievements of others mean nothing. You are not in competition with anyone but yourself.

What do the sentences above mean to you?

Write your forward journal entry.

Write as today's journal entry what your best version of yourself would say about competing with the you who showed up today.

Week 52 + 1

Happy New Year

Good Day, Journal,

Happy New Year! I want to say new year, new me, but not only would I just be making a cliché statement, but I would also be doing little more than stating the obvious. Yes, I am a new me, not because it is a new year but because each day when we awake, the present the gift to live in the moment is the Creator's way of telling us that we are reborn.

Thus, as I understand, waking each day is a rebirth, a new chance to do more than I did yesterday. Rising each morning is a fresh opportunity for reincarnation, if you will, leaving the old me behind to bring forth a new and better version. A new day is as a new year as daily the Source restores my mind, body, and soul so that it may operate on the Most Favorable' s wavelength.

Yes, Happy New Year, but each day is a happy new you, or at least it should be. And while I am delighted, of course, to be alive to see the calendar turn again to bring forth a new year, I am equally anxious.

Because each January 1st carries with it the promises of our best 365 days yet, now the task we all receive is to carry out our best-laid plans. Manifesting our worthiest dreams. Aspirations that few are willing to imagine. Envisioned projects that most folks too often abandon before Valentine's Day as they have no idea the significance of first learning to love oneself.

The New Year is also a reminder of just how much pressure there is to replicate last year's successes. The start of the forthcoming years is a heads-up to advance all the things I imagine, which I have yet to make manifest. For example, people wonder, he wrote a book last year that appeared on the New York Times bestsellers list and stayed at number one for 20 weeks; what will he do this year.

Journey Forward:

You know that you live in a "what have you done for me lately" society. But, sadly, even you subject yourself to a worse and greater misery as the questions about how you will surpass last year's achievements are not solely external.

Yes, as the year begins coming to an end, I feel the uneasiness churning in my gut. From December 25th through one minute before the bewitching hour on December 31st, I hear the doubt playing in surround sound in my mind. Blaring uncertainty about whether I can do it again, repeat this year's accomplishments next year.

Last year, you helped, served, and made sure that others knew their life mattered for at least some period. Now the quest this year is to support and provide for more people than last year. The challenge before you now is to make sure numerous others know their life matters beyond a brief introduction or encounter with you.

And let us not forget the pain in the ass condition associated with fame and fortune. Each year I am forced to remind myself that this is the life I asked the Universe to deliver unto me. After all, I am the one who pleaded and dreamed for this life. Without a doubt, I'm the one who spent the bulk of my time and energy working to prove myself worthy of the title of Internationally Renowned Public Intellectual and Humanity Propulsion Engineer.

I suppose that is why I think of my life a bit like the old Toyota commercial, "You asked for it, you got it, Toyota!" I asked to be in excellent health, to possesses abundant wealth, to share timeless wisdom. What is more, thanks to the Spirit, I am what I asked to be, and the cup of the wonders of my best life runneth over.

I am indeed living my life just as I always imagined. But at the same time, I also carry the burdens of one expected to produce considerably. Sometimes I shoulder the untenable challenge of being there for others, having some value for which others can count, and coming up with something that the masses deem worthy of sharing.

A burden that I must confess I did not take into complete consideration when I was crying out to the Heavens for a new me in a new year-long ago. I do not like people, yet my new life requires me to spend all my time and energy in others' service. I do not like people, and still, I find it impossible, thanks to my new life, to escape the burning inside demanding that I help others. Even when every fiber in my body tells me to run far away from people, the Universe commands me to do otherwise.

I am a natural loner, and now this life that I have chosen leads me to a place where I am alone now more than ever. Increasingly even when I am with others, I find myself unnaturally alone. No matter the company's location, my mind drifts to a place where others dare not go. I reside isolated perpetually in intellectual, emotional, and spiritual solitude.

Regardless of who professes to genuinely love and adore me authentically, I'm nearly always alone. My constant thoughts about what "could and must be" strengthen the grounds of those I love and adore to wish I were not present. It is not that they yearn for me to be gone from the face of the earth. They merely want me to stop thinking and questioning the meaning and purpose of life so often.

Yet to stop thinking and questioning is to be gone to another world; it is to be dead while I yet live. And thus, rather than live dead in the presence of others, even those I love and adore, I purposely choose to live as I do these days entirely alone.

So Happy New Year or is it the same day as yesterday. Is this just Groundhog Day a couple of months early? A new year with the same daily Spiritual call. Happy New Year, well, we'll see about that.

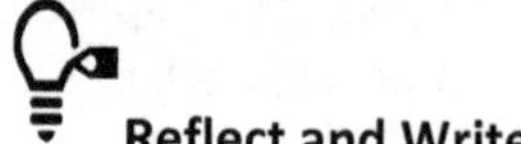

Reflect and Write:

"Yes, I am a new me, not because it is a new year but because each day when we awake, the present the gift to live in the moment is the Creator's way of telling us that we are reborn."

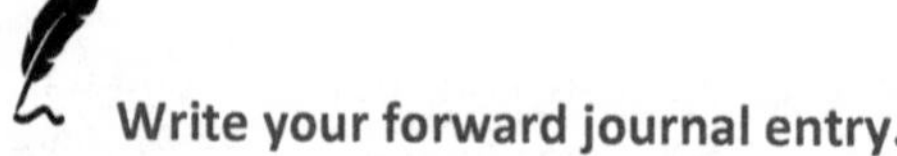

Write your forward journal entry.

Contemplate and then capture in writing what the "new you" will say to the present you in the new year!

Week 52 + 2

Commit Today

Good day Journal,

Come on, take it off! Don't be bashful now. Stop trying to act all brand new. Take them all off.

That is right, strip off every piece. Yes, socks and underwear too! Now, we're talking. Get butt ass naked.

Now, if you do not like what you see, well, you know whose fault that is. Now turn towards the mirror and take a good long look. Oh, no, don't try to divert your gaze now. It's too late for that.

Look straight ahead. Scrutinize every inch. Do you like what you see? Do you love who is standing before you? Is this the version of you, you'd want the world to see if we were capturing your nude image for posterity?

Yeah, I know, "I love me some me!" I have heard that quote for a long time. But I wonder if loving you some you include the requirement that there must be more of you to love. Somehow, I don't think more is part of this deal. I trust that concerning your weight, the absolute truth is less is more.

Check this out. Speaking of truth, I am going to keep it wholly honest with you. You are not living honorably right now. You are dishonoring the incredible Temple the Creator loaned to you. You are currently making a mockery of the Creator's exclusive gift to you.

Daily, you repeat, "I'm one hundred seventy-eight pounds of twisted steel with young Denzel chocolate sex appeal." However, the scale does not lie. Your mirror, which displays how easy it would be to pinch at least an inch of 'Grade A' fat on your waist and other areas on your body, concurs with your scale. You are a liar, a charlatan, a phony. You are not who you say you are.

One-hundred and eighty-three pounds are not 178 pounds. You just as well might go ahead and invert the numbers to read 318, 381, 813, or 831 instead of 183. From my vantage point, it does not matter. What matters is that you are not 178 pounds. Therefore, you are not only a liar. You are the overweight liar in the house.

I do not want to hear this close stuff either. Close only works in horseshoes and darts. A throw close to the center still gets you points in darts, even if it is not a bullseye. In horseshoes, a throw nearer than your opponent's toss brings you a win. But everything else being close gets you nothing.

Even the ridiculous belief that being close with a hand grenade means something is inaccurate. If you throw a hand grenade at your enemy and miss them no matter how close you still miss, your enemy can then return fire or worse, throw a hand grenade that hits you.

So, please stop with this close nonsense. And for God's sake, stop with the erroneous thinking that looking better than your peers fully dressed, I might add, means anything. Because if your peers saw you naked, they would know the truth, naked does not lie, but you and your clothes sure do.

You know what comes next, the reminder that today is a new day. Today can be the first day on the road to recovery on the return journey to be the best-naked version of yourself.

If you are willing to step up to the plate and push away from the breakfast, lunch, and dinner plates simultaneously, you should only accept the mission. You can get back to that one hundred seventy-eight pounds of twisted steel with young Denzel chocolate sex appeal. If not, you can keep doing what you have been doing, putting on weight slowly, gradually becoming who you professed you did not want to be.

I am hoping you choose to live authentically. Either be 178 pounds with ten percent or less body fat or develop a new cute phrase to tell others about your latest commitment to live a life far less than in your best health.

That is right. I'm calling you out just like your waistline on those pants is calling on you to let the waist out or get another pair of pants that is a waist size larger. Because right now, your waistline is struggling to breathe in those pants constructed for someone 178 pounds of twisted steel with young Denzel sex appeal, not for a round mound fitness hypocrite the likes of you.

Your commitment to your health is essential. I thought you knew that. The first part of the triumvirate of your daily mantra is excellent health. So, you know there is no way you can be the best version of yourself in poor health.

And yes, I know we are only talking about a couple of pounds, which, to be precise, is, in fact, more than a couple or a few. We are talking about five pounds.

But do you know what happens after gaining five pounds? First, you put on ten, then fifteen, and then do what the masses do, buying and wearing more oversized clothes. Next, you'll try to hide that underneath the baggy, larger-sized clothing is someone other than the best version of yourself—a person you would not want others to see naked.

Therefore, do yourself a huge favor today, like the size of the snacks you've been irresponsibly consuming lately. Lose the weight already, please!

I know you cannot drop every pound immediately, but you can get your act together directly. It would be best if you got your overweight lying act together right now.

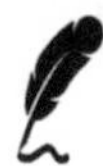

Write your forward journal entry.

Now journal forward. Let today's journal entry reflect your ideal health and what you are willing to commit to so that you can be the best version of yourself!

Week 52 + 3

Don't Waste Your Time

Good day Journal,

Do not waste your time. Do not waste your time because you do not have any time to waste.

Do you know how much time you have left? Has the Universe guaranteed you a timeline of which I am unaware? I did not think so. So, you do not know how much time you have left after all, do you? Then let me repeat, you do not have time to waste.

In life, you are not here today, gone tomorrow. In this life, the only life, you are here today, gone today. That is how life works, truly. As the 'Elements' attested melodically in 1975, ♪That's the way (yaow!) Of the world (yaow! Hey, yeah!) ♪.[xiii]

I tell you not to waste your time because I love you. Instead, I implore you to pay attention to using each precious second that the Source gifts.

It is finally time to do what is in your best interest. It is past time that you performed an audit of your time. It is time to take an in-depth analysis of 5 Ws and 1 H of your life.

Now is the time to examine the who, what, where, when, why, and how you spend your time. In this very moment, you need to determine if your undeserved finite time gets applied to living the life you always imagined. Or if you are wasting the unmerited limited moments on yesterday's history, a preceding that leads to tomorrow's regret.

As if you were a DJ and the Universe was calling into your radio station to make a song request, play some 'Bone Thugs and Harmony.'[xiv] Live out one of their most important messages.

Journey Forward:

♪ Wake up, wake up, wake up; it's the 1st of the month.
To get up, get up, get up, so cash your checks and get up. ♪

Yes, I know it is not the first of the month, really, but the "first of the month" provides sound symbolism. What is crucial is for you to accept you have no time to waste today. You should approach today as though this is the first of the month, an exciting day, perhaps the best day of the month for one struggling financially.

It is the first of the month when the most precious marginalized folks usually get paid. The first of the month is when the social system provides a temporary net to catch us. For many, it's the short respite when one can finally breathe again if only catching a break to exhale for a second or two. This first of the month analogy should be your approach to life daily.

Breath in today and every day as if it is undoubtedly the first and best day of not the month but of your life. Live today and each day with the unmatched vigor and urgency of one rushing to cash their check at the first of the month.

Because as I tell you repeatedly today, this very moment could be the last day you get. Today could not only be the first of the month; it could be the last day of your life. Thus, I'll keep beating the same old drum, playing the same old song. While you are here, you have no time to waste.

As you audit the time of your life, please take a moment to note who steals time from you. Who are they who not only waste their graciously gifted time but steal yours too?

Be wary of those who will not do what is best for their life but want to rob you of the limited time to live up to your potential. It would be best if you did not allow others to use and abuse you. Do not waste irreplaceable time. Do not squander one-off moments donated benevolently to you by the Spirit.

What things are you doing daily that waste your time? How often are you checking your phone, looking at email, and social media? Take an accounting.

How often do inanimate objects rob you of consciously living? How frequently do nonliving things deprive you of the vivacious now? Note how much time you spend reading and obsessing over another's life rather than being present? How frequently have you circumvented meaningful personal relationships by not being fully present to experience the entirety of your life right here at this moment?

Where is your time being used? Is it being used in a place where you are creating your best life, or is it being wasted in areas that are monuments to nothingness? Where do you want your life to go? If you are not there, if you are not on your way to where you have always wanted to be, you have likely been wasting time.

When will you get it together? When will you get a clue that this life, your only life, belongs to you and you alone? When will you commit totally? I mean an elbow-to-asshole working day and night commitment to be the best version of yourself possible?

Will you finally do it today? Or will you put it off foolishly for some indeterminate time? Will you continue to delay for some unpromised future moment?

Why are you wasting time? Do you know? Do you know? Do you know? Money, I know it's not the shoes. But I would like you to discover soon why you will not give all you have within you all the time, which you now have available to live up to your God-given potential.

How do you want others to remember you when your time is up? Will you merely be one with great opportunities lost? Shall you be the one with massive unrealized potential? Or will you utilize the gifted time to fulfill the mission: to help, serve, and make sure others know their life matters.

You are very nearly out of time. I know it. I can feel it way deep down in my soul. You have no time to waste.

Please, I am begging you on bended knee. Do not waste your time!

Reflect and Write:

It’s the third week of the new year. It’s time again to journal forward.

Journey Forward:

Write what your life will look like when you start making the most of every minute of this year. Be specific. Give concrete examples.

Works Cited

Anderson, S., Brown, C., Wilson, D., Harris II, J., & Lewis, T. (2011). My Last [Recorded by B. Sean, & C. Brown]. West Hollywood, CA, USA.

Burns, R. (1995). *Auld Lang Syne.* Scots Musical Museum.

Dr. Martin Luther King, J. (1960, April 10). If You Can't Fly, Then Run. *Keep Moving from This Mountain*. Atlanta, GA, USA: Spelman College Museum.

James, K. (1993). *The Original African Heritage Study Bible.* (P. The Reverend Cain Hope Felder, Ed.) Nashville, Tennessee, USA: The James C. Winston Publishing Company.

Longfellow, H. W. (n.d.). The Legend Beautiful. *The Atlantic.*

McCane, B., U-Neek, D., Powell, M., Bone, W., Bone, L., & Bone, K. (1994). 1st of tha Month [Recorded by B. Thugs-n-Harmony]. Los Angeles, CA, USA.

Nelson, P. R. (1982). Gigolos Get Lonely Too [Recorded by T. Time]. On *What Time Is It?* Los Angeles, CA, USA.

Nelson, P. R., & Dickerson, D. (1981). Cool (Part 2) [Recorded by T. Time]. Minneapolis, MN, USA.

Schmidlin, C., Townsend, R., Ampah, K., Jones, L. C. (Producers), Townsend, R. (Writer), & Townsend, R. (Director). (1991). *The Five Heartbeats* [Motion Picture]. 20th Century Fox.

White, M., Stepney, C., & White, V. (1974). That's the Way of the World [Recorded by W. &. Earth]. New York City, New York, USA.

Notes

[i] (James, 1993)
[ii] (James, 1993)
[iii] (Burns, 1995)
[iv] (Nelson, Gigolos Get Lonely Too, 1982)
[v] (Nelson & Dickerson, Cool (Part 2), 1981)
[vi] (James, 1993)
[vii] (James, 1993)
[viii] (Longfellow)
[ix] (James, 1993)
[x] (Dr. Martin Luther King, 1960)
[xi] (Anderson, Brown, Wilson, Harris II, & Lewis, 2011)
[xii] (Schmidlin, Townsend, Ampah, & Jones, 1991)
[xiii] (White, Stepney, & White, 1974)
[xiv] (McCane, et al., 1994)

CPSIA information can be obtained
at www.ICGtesting.com
Printed in the USA
LVHW030744100921
697444LV00005B/392